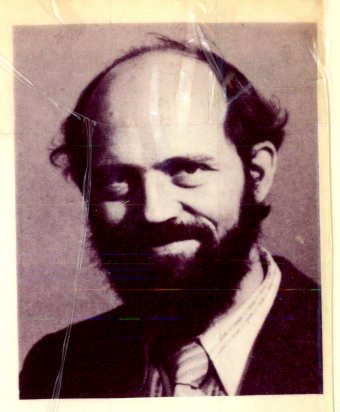

Alfred P. French, M.D., is currently an Assistant Professor of Child Psychiatry at the University of California, Davis, and the Sacramento Medical Center, where he was a Resident in Psychiatry and a Child Fellow. Dr. French received his B.A. degree in biology from Carleton College, an M.A. in biochemistry and an M.D. from the University of Kansas, and completed his internship in internal medicine at the University of Iowa.

DISTURBED CHILDREN AND THEIR FAMILIES

Innovations in Evaluation and Treatment

Alfred P. French, M.D.

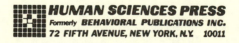

HUMAN SCIENCES PRESS
Formerly *BEHAVIORAL PUBLICATIONS INC.*
72 FIFTH AVENUE, NEW YORK, N.Y. 10011

Library of Congress Catalog Number 75-11003

ISBN: 0-87705-263-8

Printed in the United States of America
789 987654321

Library of Congress Cataloging in Publication Data
French, Alfred P
     Disturbed children and their families.

     (Child psychiatry and psychology series)
     Bibliography: p.
     Includes index.
     1. Child psychiatry.   2. Family psychotherapy.
I. Reid, Gerri Wold. II. Title. [DNLM: 1. Mental disorders—In infancy and childhood. WS350 F873d]
RJ499.F77   618.9'28'915   75-11003
ISBN 0-87705-263-8

CONTENTS

This book is dedicated to all my teachers, the most important of whom are my patients.

INTRODUCTION

By Irving Berlin, M.D.*

It is very heartening to read this book by a young child psychiatrist. Youth is not imprisoned by tradition. Dr. French's thinking is fresh and uncontaminated by dogma. Several of his ideas which are vital to the thrust of this book are the genuine gold of new discoveries. For the record, the tradition of child psychiatrists working exclusively with the child and social workers with the parents has been abandoned in many training settings well over a decade ago. Other historical and clinical inaccuracies are trivial when compared to this fresh approach to viewing the evaluation and treatment of children and their families in new and creative contexts.

The value of this book is that it couples the theory of a systems and structural approach to family therapy with an integration of a method of systematic evaluation which focuses on developmental phenomenae and stress as important variables in assessing the child and each family member to reach a viable, dynamic formulation of problems as well as strengths and diagnostic possibilities.

*Professor of Psychiatry and Pediatrics, Vice-Chairman for Child Mental Health, University of California, Davis, School of Medicine at the Sacramento Medical Center; President, American Academy of Child Psychiatry.

To me of great interest was Dr. French's new and very effective way of conceptualizing both problems and strengths in a family. This method, which Dr. French calls a four-item or four-place system, is an innovative and effective method of viewing diagnosis and therapeutic process.

Evaluation of the family in terms of its total anxiety—who is the most anxious, who carries the symptoms in the family, the family's capacity for change, who in it is most capable of change, and who carries the power in the family—provides an innovative and very useful method of evaluation and constant reassessment of family dynamics. One can understand not only what is happening in the family but also what the alternative roles of the therapist might be. The method provides signals to the therapist of potentially effective and harmful interventions in family therapy.

Coupled with this delightfully new and effective model is a very thorough outline for evaluation of children and families. Of enormous value are numerous case examples to illustrate every step of evaluation and integration of data which makes up most of the work. The two long examples of Dr. French's new concept of family interaction provide excellent illustrations of how the model works.

This is indeed a text for all trainees and most workers in family and child therapy. It happily combines a modern scientific approach to family therapy both in theory and in practice, a rare combination. I could only hope that all of us would learn and teach such a thorough and systematic approach to evaluation. Only a child psychiatrist as bright, as young, and as adventuresome a thinker would have attempted and succeeded in writing so useful and challenging a text in child and family evaluation and treatment.

PREFACE

The development of a child-family psychiatrist includes many transitions: from biology to the "hard" sciences and back again, from biology to pathology, from basic sciences to the practice of medicine, from biological medicine to psychiatry, and, finally, from "child" psychiatry to a hybrid state where we range freely from the biological level through the psychological and family levels to the social and institutional levels. But the task is always the same: how, in a complex system, can we make the most beneficial change with the least effort and risk?

Among these transitions, the last was most difficult for me because families presented terrible and painful problems, and the lack of structure in assessment, formulation, and treatment was frightening.

One day Dr. Marge Steward, a supervisor, said: "The behavior of that family may be difficult and confusing, but behavior is never *random.*" A light dawned. The family (including each individual member's unique biological contribution) became an organized system, and in that context, the child's symptoms made some sense. I shifted from despair to excitement. Papers by Framo (1970), Bowen (1966), and Thomas, Chess, and Birch (1970) as well as books by Minuchin (1974) and Satir (1967) held out the hope that the rules underlying the clinical chaos could be understood well enough for clinicians to construct a formulation and treatment plan based on immediate clinical data. Forrester (1968) offered another ray of hope by demonstrating that a structurally simple system can exhibit extremely complex behavior; i.e., it can oscillate. Therefore, it was reasonable (or at least possible) to hope that, conversely, complex behavior might be a reflection of a structurally simple system. In other words, a troubled family might have one problem at the level of its structural rules rather than the innumerable problems it presented to the clinician. The clinical payoff of these speculations was immediate. My anxiety and sense of helplessness about working with families shifted toward an interest in learning with them about the complex interplay of factors that created and maintained their symptoms. And, most important, the families improved.

Over a period of time, my interest in the problem of evaluating the symptomatic child-family system led to this book, which provides tools that fellow explorers can use as a map and compass to guide them into the same terrain.

At present, an active and often acrimonious debate is going on within child psychiatry. On the one hand, there is the traditional child-guidance approach, which in general advocates that the most symptomatic member of the family (in this book called the "identified patient") should be seen by the primary clinician, preferably a psychiatrist, while the parents are seen by a social worker. The other point of view is represented by the growing number of family therapists who, in general, advocate that the entire family as a unit or system, rather than the identified patient alone, should be the primary focus. As is often the case, vigorous debate in an area that is high in anxiety and low in good data and conceptual models tends to deteriorate into accusations and counteraccusations. This is occurring in the field of child psychiatry at the present time, as McDermott and Char (1974) outlined in a paper with the intriguing title "The Undeclared War Between Child and Family Therapy."

Because he who pitches his tent in the midst of a raging battlefield is well advised to clarify his position, I will outline the bias of this book at the outset. It is sometimes best to see the identified patient alone and focus on the interaction between patient and therapist. In this case it makes sense for the parents to be seen, if at all, by another therapist. There are situations, however, where it is best to see the entire family together, making the *family system* the primary focus of therapy. This book is about the evaluation that should *precede* the selection of a therapeutic approach in a particular case. Elegant therapy—whether of a child or of a family—that is based on a poor formulation is a house built on sand. Through the development of increasingly powerful clinical tools, I hope that we will be able to offer specific, well-founded opinions about which specific modality of treatment, if any, is indicated in a particular case.

I would like to comment on the hallowed tradition in child psychiatry and social work that the psychiatrist should see the identified patient while a social worker sees the parents or other family members. In my opinion, this tradition is something of a sacred cow, and I would like to share my fantasies about the theoretical basis for it. Medical historians have observed that the fundamental model of disease which has long prevailed is in essence a "demon theory": in other words, disease occurs because a person is beset by some evil influence from the outside (Inglis, 1965). In pneumonia, for instance, the evil influence is a bacterium or virus, which creates the signs and symptoms of pneumonia. In behavioral disorders in children, the phenomenon is somewhat more complex but usually can be reduced to the same theoretical model: the child is essentially healthy unless an outside influence (e.g., bad parenting in the case of nurture or bad genes in the case of nature) generates a conflict that functions the way a germ does in an infectious disease or as a demon did in an earlier model. But to return to the point, psychiatrists seem to believe, deep in their physician's hearts (and social workers, by compliance, state behavioral agreement), that somewhere within the symptomatic child's mind there dwells, in one form or another, a demon and that this demon must be removed by appropriate ritual. The more frightening the symptoms, the more frightening the demon, and the more impressive must be the priest who will contend with it. In short, the priest with the greatest number of raiments (the psychiatrist) deals with the most threatening demons, while the priest with fewer raiments (the social worker) takes on the "lesser" task of coping with the parents. (In Chapter 8 I will argue that the social worker's task in this situation is in fact the more difficult one.) I present this fantasy quite seriously. Although I am not opposed to parallel therapy in some cases, I can find no solid rationale for the tradition that the physician should see the identified patient while the social worker sees the parents. In my opinion, the most suitable therapeutic modality and specific assignment of therapist or therapists should remain an open question until a reasonable evaluation of the individual case has been completed.

Writing this book has been fun and without doubt the most important educational experience of my life. The evaluative outline with which I began has led me on an ever widening search for conceptual clarity and clinical utility. In its present form, the outline serves as the framework for Chapters 3 through 7. In Chapter 9, it appears in abbreviated form as a list of tools for everyday use. At this point, I urge you to stop reading and write your own outline for evaluating a child-family problem. By doing so, you will learn far more than I could ever teach you about the matter.

I hope that this book will be theoretically challenging, clinically useful, and, above all, make your work with children and families easier, more effective, and more enjoyable.

The staff of the East Sacramento Mental Health Center were an invaluable resource during field trials of the evaluation format presented in the Appendix as well as its many precursors. I offer special thanks to Andrea Lambert, R.N., M.S., and JoAnn Fallow, R.N., M.S., for their willingness to try new clinical tools.

I also gratefully acknowledge the help of Dr. Baruch Fischoff, of the Oregon Research Institute, who provided essential ideas and references for the sections on formulation in Chapters 2 and 7, and Drs. Joe Tupin and Don Langsley, who offered encouragement and advice at many points during the project's development. My special thanks to Drs. Marge Steward and Larry Greenberg for their inspired teaching.

Finally, my thanks to Norma Fox, editor-in-chief of Human Sciences Press, through whose efforts this book was published. The editing was done by Elizabeth Bowman, who reorganized into readable form my original unwieldy manuscript. Gerri Wold Reid provided the cartoons; Kathryn Marr was responsible for the technical illustrations. The manuscript was typed by Louise Johansson and Marcia Wendt.

Chapter 1

THE FAMILY AS A SYSTEM

The theoretical issues underlying this book are as old as the debate between Parmenides, who claimed that change was an illusion and that "the world is one," and Heraclitus, who insisted that only change is real: "We can never step in the same river twice because it is always changing."

This debate, like all apparently unresolvable paradoxes, has led to a deeper understanding of reality than either approach alone could provide. Current efforts to include both change and permanence as primary realities include general system theory and structuralism (see Piaget, 1971; von Bertalanffy, 1968). I will outline these conceptual tools and then attempt to use their problem-solving power to attack the following clinical paradox: How can a family simultaneously love and damage a child?

THE NEW WORLD VIEW

We are in the midst of a major revolution. The past few decades have seen such profound changes throughout the arts and sciences that no fundamental concept of under-standing has been left untouched. We are experiencing nothing less than a major revision in the nature of Western consciousness. The world view of the past 2,000 years—resting on the logic of Aristotle, the mathematics of Euclid, and the physics of Newton—described the world as a fixed and static entity. Thus a complete description of all initial conditions was theoretically adequate to predict events at any subsequent point in time. The polarity between the static form and the ongoing process as a primary locus of reality is as old as Western philosophy itself (Stallknecht & Brumbaugh, 1950).

In recent times, however, world view that emphasizes relationship rather than states has emerged. (Capek, 1961; Reusch, 1953). The physics of Galileo introduced the con-cept of the field; the mathematics of Lobachevski demon-strated that there are several internally consistent mathematical systems, of which Euclidean geometry is only one; and the physics of Einstein demonstrated that al-though mass varies with velocity, the speed of light is al-ways constant with respect to an observer. In his summary of this revolution, Buckley stated that our primary focus has shifted from *material substance* to *organization*. Therefore, there has been

> a shift from statics, structure, somativity and one-way causal-ity to dynamics, process, emergence, and complex mutual interactions and feedback cycles. It is not the nature of the parts alone that are basic to any whole, but the way that they are interrelated that gives them their characteristic proper-ties . . . The parts may come to take on properties that they owe specifically to being parts of a larger whole [1968, p. xxiv, italics added].

In short, the old world view was essentially that the world was a closed system in which nothing could be genuinely new; the current world view is that the universe is an open system in which genuine novelty is a real possibility.[1]

The classical world view could account for closed but not open systems, and despite its astounding success in the realm of physics, it could not handle problems raised in biology and the behavioral sciences. Thus a crisis occurred as science was forced to develop a conceptual model that was adequate to deal with open systems. As Ludwig von Bertalanffy, the father of general systems theory, stated:

> It is a change in basic categories of thought of which the complexities of modern technology are only one . . . mani-festation. In one way or another, we are forced to deal with complexities, with "wholes" or "systems", in all fields of knowledge. This implies a basic re-orientation in scientific thinking [1968, p. 5].

In other words, the organism is capable of modifying itself and its environment continuously through interactions with that environment. This is a heady concept for the child psychiatrist! If we take the systems view seriously, we can no longer be satisfied with a simple diagnosis; we must seek a formulation that considers the importance of all family members and their interactions. Gone forever are simplistic "explanations" such as bad genes or bad parenting. The systems view requires a statement that takes the following general form: The child and family have interacted in such a way that the symptomatic behaviors have emerged as a reasonable solution to developmental and life problems and opportunities as the family experienced them. To this we must add something about the reversibility or irreversibility of these behaviors.

Are we then tossed into a chaotic state in which relativism means lack of order and any statement is as good as any other? Fortunately, this is not the case; the emphasis is simply shifted from a description of states to an emphasis on relationships. As von Bertalanffy pointed out: "The basis of the open system model is the dynamic interaction of its components [1968, p. 150].

Over the past ten years, the literature about families has been organized increasingly around the concept of the family as a system to emphasize the relationships between all family members (Bowen, 1966; Framo, 1970; Haley, 1964; Minuchin, 1974; Satir, 1971). The objective of this chapter is to outline the fields of general system theory and structuralism and to discuss some of the implications of these theoretical advances for child and family psychiatry.

GENERAL SYSTEMS THEORY AND STRUCTURALISM

The field of general systems theory developed by von Bertalanffy (1968) is a direct response to the challenge of the open system. To summarize our earlier discussion: general systems theory seeks to deal with systems that are capable of continuous internal modification over time as opposed to aggregates that are, in theory at least, predictable in their behavior.

A system can be defined as a structure composed of a set of elements and a set of rules that specify the relationship among the elements (Forrester, 1968; Gray & Rizzo, 1969; Hall & Fagen, 1968; von Bertalanffy, 1968). Piaget defined structure in somewhat more mathematical and abstract terms as a "system of transformations. In short, the notion of structure is comprised of three key ideas: the idea of wholeness, the idea of transformation, and the idea of self-regulation [1970, p. 5]." Systems maintain their integrity through the use of feedback loops—arrangements of components that serve to move information from consequence to decision-maker, thus permitting the organism to correct deviations and stay on course.

Physically, systems consist of hierarchically nested subsystems—e.g., cells, tissues, organs, organ systems, individual organisms—which are themselves ultimately composed of feedback loops. The physical structure of the system must provide for (1) communication, (2) regulation of critical parameters so that those parameters will not be too far above or below permitted levels, and (3) change of the reference points with respect to which the feedback loops operate.

Functionally, a system must be capable of (1) maintaining homeostasis—sustaining a relatively steady state despite the continuous flow of both matter and energy through the system, (2) changing the reference norms with respect to which homeostasis occurs, and (3) deciding which of these two basic modes of functioning should be used. The first function, homeostatic processes, maintains the constant state of the organism while modifying part of the environment; the second results in a fundamental modification of the organism itself as it responds to the environment. Piaget defined homeostasis as assimilation and the shift in the basic reference structure with respect to which the organism maintains homeostasis as accommodation (Piaget, 1971; Piaget & Inhelder, 1969). Adaptation can be defined as the balance between assimilation, or homeostatic processes, on the one hand, and accommodation, or shifts in the basic nature of the organism itself, on the other. In the human, the ego selects the appropriate balance between the two (French & Steward, 1975).

In this book the following terms will be used for these functions:

- *Type I process* (homeostasis or assimilation). Type I processes are defined as all functions involved in maintaining the steady state of an open system operating with respect to a fixed set of reference points.

- *Type II process* (accommodation). Type II processes are defined as shifts in the fundamental reference structure with respect to which the organism maintains its homeostatic balance.
- *Adaptation.* Adaptation is the result of Type I processes (assimilation, homeostasis) and Type II processes (accommodation).

These distinctions are enormously useful when handling clinical problems. In general, Type I processes occur rapidly and easily and are always the strategies of choice when a problem arises. Type II processes occur slowly and with difficulty and are considered only after all reasonable Type I options have been exhausted.

Developing parallel to systems theory, structuralism evolved a similar conceptual model from a somewhat different base. The initial impetus for the development of structuralism was the attempt to cope with the dilemmas of evolution (Piaget, 1963). The general concepts of structuralism and systems theory are similar, but those of structuralism are somewhat more abstract: "A structure is a system with a set of laws . . . laws of transformation. A given structure is characterized by the type of transformation which its laws represent. . . . They are self-regulating; there is a sort of closure [Piaget, 1972, p. 15]." With structuralism, Piaget presented his answer to the ancient nature-nurture controversy. Although some of his colleagues view him as a maturationist (one who proposes that development is only a matter of maturation of the nervous system) and others view him as a neobehaviorist (one who proposes that intellectual development results simply from the impress of events on the mind), Piaget insists that he is an interactionist:

What interests me is the creation of new thoughts that are not preformed, not predetermined by nervous system maturation, nor predetermined by encounter with the environment but are constructed within the individual himself, constructed internally through the process of reflexive abstraction and constructed externally through the process of experience [1972, p. 25].

Thus our concern is the growing, developing child who, through experience, actively creates an understanding of the world.

Beckett (1973) cautioned that applying general systems theory to behavior would not necessarily be easy, that we must consciously avoid putting the "new wine" of systems theory into the "old wine skins" of what is essentially a closed-system model:

> The idea of *systems as sets of smaller wholes* and the idea of the *larger wholes themselves,* are both capable of being seen as parts and pieces, with all the limitations of atomistic thinking. . . . Certainly there is no great conceptual leap for mankind here. . . . [However,] the concepts of *interrelationships* and of *dynamism* which are the corollaries of the concepts of systems and wholism are key ideas of general systems theory . . . [p. 296 –297].

In other words, to realize the full power of the concept of the family as a system, we must look carefully at our formulations of family dynamics to make certain that we are not using the new "systems" language while thinking in terms of a closed model.

Commoner (1971) has summarized the concepts of general systems theory into four useful rules: (1) everything is connected to everything else, (2) everything has to go somewhere, (3) nature knows best, and (4) there is no free lunch. To make his rules more amenable to clinical work, we might paraphrase them as follows:

1. Everyone in a family is important.
2. Unresolved tensions will always be expressed somewhere at some time, possibly in a highly disguised form: i.e., problems cannot be swept under the rug.

3. The family (and every individual in it) has its own internal wisdom. There are reasons for any persistent pattern of behavior, no matter how "sick" or symptomatic. Therefore, the clinician is well advised to learn as much as possible about the family rules before seeking to facilitate change.

4. Families that try to resolve one problem by balancing it off against another do not achieve a free solution to either problem; on the contrary, they may drastically reduce their degrees of freedom in the future.

THE CHALLENGE OF CLINICAL APPLICATION

Now that we have a general outline of the concepts of system and structure, let us look at the family in these terms. In this book, the word family means all individuals who are a stable part of our index individual's social environment, especially those who exert a significant influence on his development and on his belief structure, including the rules of change. (Our index individual, of course, is the symptomatic child, or identified patient.) The term family will be used in these functional terms without confining the discussion to the current (or past) living unit. Operationally, this means that anyone whose feelings or opinions are or have been of special importance to the family should be included in the family tree.

According to our definition of system, the family is composed of a set of elements and a set of rules that determine the relationships among elements and function in a way that makes the whole greater than the sum of its parts in at least one dimension. Furthermore, structuralism's immense problem-solving power can be brought to bear on family problems since the family, like the formal structure, is characterized by (1) wholeness (the whole is greater than the sum of its parts), (2) transformation (it remains a stable entity despite the fact that individuals within it are continually changing according to an orderly process defined by family rules), and (3) self-regulation (it maintains order during change).

How do we translate the jargon of systems theory into clinical work with families? The time-honored concept of the collective mythology, or belief structure, provides one useful clue. The belief structure provides the roles for each family member, communication occurs between all family members, and family rules provide the means for correcting excessive deviation from family norms. In other words, the family belief structure provides the reference system with respect to which family homeostasis occurs. Therefore, the family belief structure is as essential to the functioning of the family organism as physiological reference points are to the functioning of the body (Ferreira, 1963). If the body has no reference point for blood sugar, the result is diabetes. The same kind of "metabolic" chaos results in the family when reference points are unavailable or unclear. According to the terms defined earlier, this can be conceptualized as a Type II problem: that is, a process involving the system's reference points. When a reference point is clear but cannot be maintained, the result is anxiety or panic. A parallel state occurs in the body when the blood oxygen cannot be held at an adequate level. This is a Type I problem: that is, it is impossible for the family to maintain homeostasis despite the presence of a reference point. Similarly, the family will experience chaos if its reference system—i.e., its mythology—is unclear (Type II problem) and anxiety or panic if its members cannot approximate the roles required by the family mythology (Type I problem).

Again and again, we observe the incredible tenacity with which a family will support the collective mythology, and we are amazed at how vigorously a family will struggle to hold family members in their roles while simultaneously complaining about some of the behaviors those roles require! If we view this behavior as an arbitrarily willful effort on the family's part to avoid change or if we infer that the family enjoys the symptomatic child's (or belabored therapist's) plight, our only options are disappointment, frustration, and anger. If, on the other hand, we recognize what is involved when we ask a family to shift its reference points —if we recognize that we are asking it to change the very reality of its world—we may feel less irritated by what we experience clinically as resistance. (Later, I will discuss in detail the family's capacity to shift its reference points—i.e., carry out a successful Type II process—as a clinically critical parameter of family function.) Only the family can judge the cost of a fundamental shift in the rules and belief system that provide the foundation of its existence. The first responsibility of any organism is to protect its reference system because without that system, there is total chaos. Resistance, in other words, may be a reflection of profound wisdom!

In summary, the family can be perceived as an open system that maintains a relatively constant steady state despite the continuous flow of energy and material through the system. It does so by maintaining communication from consequences to decision points; a hierarchical nesting of these feedback loops makes the system extremely stable.

The family belief structure, or mythology, provides the reference points with respect to which corrective decisions are made. The family rules not only reflect the content of this mythology but include the criteria for changing the rules and the means for correcting deviations from role-appropriate behavior. Correction of these deviations with respect to constant reference points is homeostasis (Type I process). A shift in the reference points themselves, with respect to which homeostasis occurs, is accommodation (Type II process). The end result of the two processes is *adaptation*.

SYSTEMS AND SYMPTOMS

Our theoretical discussion of the family as a system can now turn to a practical task. How do we conceptualize disease and symptom in a way that will be useful when working with symptomatic children and their families? The classical theory of disease, which is used to this day, is in essence a "demon" theory. The organism is sick because it has been invaded, damaged, or depleted by a foreign element or demon. In most instances, this concept of disease serves well in the field of medicine. Foreign agents such as traumas, infecting organisms, cancers, and so forth can be readily conceptualized as invading the organism from the outside, while deficiencies of vitamins and minerals create characteristic disease entities from within. Inglis noted that the basic concept of disease has been a matter of too much or not enough:

> Man is sick because there is something in his body that does not belong to it, or he is sick because something has been removed from his organism that is necessary to life. Understandably, diseases were often attributed to the malice of enemies introducing something into, or withdrawing something from the patient [1965, pp. 6–7].

Clearly, this concept of disease, which carries with it the implicit definition of a symptom as an extraneous element or an externally caused deficiency, is appropriate to the closed model of reality discussed earlier: i.e., disease is a simple matter of excess or deficiency. If the child and his family are a system, however, the parts are, to varying degrees, related to each other. In other words, Commoner's (1971) first rule that everything is connected to everything else applies. We must therefore revise at a fundamental level the concepts of disease and symptom. For example, infectious disease must be conceptualized, not simply as the presence of foreign organisms, but as a complex relationship involving both host and organism (Schopler & Luftin, 1969).

These theoretical issues are of utmost practical importance because the clinician's position in these matters will be reflected immediately in his day-to-day practice. If we conceptualize behavioral disorders of childhood as the simple result of bad parenting, we are operating within a simple demonology model and our sole option is to scapegoat the parents. Obviously, this is precisely what has occurred in an overwhelming number of cases. Parents of symptomatic children have been the victims of a mind-boggling list of accusations. The term schizophrenic mother, which is now losing favor (Schopler & Luftin, 1969; Arieti, 1974), may be the clearest example. Obviously, parenting style is a critical component of a child's environment, and the child-rearing methods of some parents are so poor that permanent damage results. The challenge is to work with these parents without becoming angry and yet remain fully aware of their (often enormous) damaging impact on the child. The practice of assigning different members of the treatment team to either the child *or* the parents may result in sweeping the problem under the rug, only to have it blossom forth in the form of conflicts between staff! At this point, we can see that there is nothing more practical than a good theory. The power of the general systems view lies in its ability to view all members of the system as involved in the creation, maintenance, and modification of all family patterns, adaptive and maladaptive, without scapegoating.

Stress

Stress can be defined as anything that moves the organism away from homeostasis for a time and with sufficient force to prohibit the organism from reestablishing balance easily. Thus a symptom is any maneuver the organism uses to compensate for this imbalance, which is quantitatively or qualitatively outside the range of normal homeostatic processes. (Menninger, Mayman & Pruyser, 1963). An organism must be able to adapt itself to disturbing forces, either by bringing the disturbance under control (assimilation) or by modifying itself to meet the new demands (accommodation).

Most families handle most stresses adaptively: that is, they find ways to respond to the stress without losing their balance. Stress often results in an increased capacity to adapt as the family system, like an individual, grows and matures in response to life's challenges. Indeed, some stress is essential for the health of any organism. But if the stress is severe or prolonged enough, the organism must resort to expensive measures to maintain balance and may never regain its previous level of functioning. In this book, our primary concern will be these latter processes, particularly those in which the family's efforts to maintain balance involve a child's symptomatic behavior.

Therefore, it is essential to differentiate between the transient stress reaction and disease. The transient stress reaction involves a *reversible* deviation from the organism's normal state: i.e., the organism returns to normal once the stress is gone. In the case of disease, undesirable changes are irreversible—the organism cannot return to its original state and its adaptability decreases. For example, it is normal and necessary for blood pressure to increase with exercise. This is a temporary, reversible, and stress-related response. But if the blood pressure does not return to normal, a disease exists and we are talking about an entirely different phenomenon. Note that disease is defined, not as the extent to which the organism's configuration deviates from normality, but the extent to which the deviation is fixed. Health and pathology may therefore be defined in terms of the organism's ability to respond in a flexible, adaptive way to the stresses that confront it, rather than in terms of any particular *configurations* the organism uses. Obviously, the more configurations the organism has at its disposal, the more adaptable it will become. Conversely, its adaptability will decrease as it loses this kind of flexibility. In other words, a healthy response to stress may result in increased adaptability and an unhealthy response, in decreased adaptability. The following discussion focuses on the unhealthy responses.

Balance Bargains

The family, like any organism, must maintain balance while minimizing the amount of energy it expends. If stressed beyond its capacity to respond adaptively and if unable to avoid the stress, a family has three options. One, it can ignore the stress. This is dangerous. Two, it can use sufficient energy to oppose the stress directly and thus maintain balance. This is expensive and exhausting. Three, it can resort to a "balance bargain"—a maneuver by which it reorganizes itself so that a force that was initially experienced as stressful is either neutralized or experienced as useful or even essential. If this maneuver was reversible and the family could return, poststress, to its initial configuration, all would be well. But balance bargains are unhealthy to the extent that they become irreversible and thus reduce the family's ability to respond adaptively to future stress. In short, the family has run afoul of the rule that there is no free lunch!

Consider an individual who must carry a heavy object. The easiest way to carry it is close to the body. But if the object smells bad, a conflict arises. One way to resolve this conflict is to carry the object at arm's length, but the individual would soon be exhausted. Another solution would be to rest his arm on a table. This balance bargain reduces the individual's output of energy, but obviously it also restricts his movements.

Placing the "new wine" of general systems thinking into the "old wine skin" of the demon model of disease, family clinicians are sometimes prone to say, in one way or another, that the family or the family system *made* the child, or identified patient sick. This conceptualization is appropriate for the simple model of disease, which states that an external agent, whether virus or family, inflicts damage on the organism. In this model, the causality is a simple linear one from family to child; replacing the term family with the term family system does not change the underlying conceptual model. Conceptualizing the family as a system, however, requires us to recognize that the identified patient and his family interact in a complex way to create and maintain the illness.

Stress, by definition, requires compromises and adjustments. By the time the family presents itself for clinical evaluation and treatment (especially when an extremely serious and chronic problem is involved), it may have learned to reduce stress by using the child's symptoms to reduce the overall energy it needs to function on a day-to-day basis. I am convinced that, in general, these balance bargains were orginally "intended," on an unconscious level, to be reversible arrangements that would permit the family to continue its daily life under conditions of stress.

Unfortunately, however, balance bargains can be hazardous. If reversibility is lost, the symptoms are locked in, and the family's ability to provide an adaptive environment for the growing child is reduced. This situation is most likely to occur when the family tries to solve two problems at once—i.e., by balancing an external stress against an internal one. For example, consider the husband and wife who feel a deep hostility toward one other and are unable to express it in a healthy way. If they have a multiply handicapped child, the situation, although painful, may provide them with the means to express their hostility toward one another. This balance bargain may be adaptive in the short run, and if we assume reversibility, it is only a harmless expedient. However, to their distress, the couple may discover in the future that (1) they indeed made such a bargain in the first place, (2) although initially intended as a temporary measure, the bargain had lost its reversibility and is now deeply embedded in the family process, and (3) they were actively, albeit covertly, attempting not only to maintain the child's difficulties but to increase them. The clinical challenge of this type of case is obvious. On the one hand, the family's involvement in maintaining the child's symptoms must be explored. On the other hand, the parents are enormously vulnerable to and become justifiably angry when confronted with any suggestion that they do not love their child. Furthermore, the clinician may well view himself as the child's defender and find overt or covert satisfaction in attacking the parents. Since this attack is, of course, on the child's "behalf," yet another balance bargain is introduced if the clinician covertly anticipates the child's gratitude for being rescued!

The fact that symptoms often become an intrinsic part of the family structure does not mean that we must scapegoat parents. The very nature of organisms does not permit the family to function otherwise if stress is severe and prolonged. Families request treatment when the balance bargains become bankrupt, as revealed by a crisis. For example, the couple with the handicapped child might eagerly and sincerely seek help when the child is unable to function in school. The clinician becomes aware that the child's symptoms represent a secondary gain for the family when the parents consistently "forget" to carry out some aspects of treatment. Commonly, of course, additional tensions may develop around the child's symptoms, and the balance bargain turns out to be a relatively ineffective means of relieving stress after all. In a useful paper titled "Symptoms from a Family Transactional Viewpoint,"

Framo discussed at length how symptoms develop and are maintained within the family.

Dystonic and Syntonic Symptoms

So far, we have discussed the family's responses to stress in fairly general terms. We will now explore two additional avenues: symptoms that push the family apart and symptoms that pull the family together. When describing these symptoms, it is convenient to use the terms syntonic and dystonic, which are commonly used in the literature and correspond readily to the conceptual model developed here. Dystonic symptoms push the family apart and are a drain on the family's energies. Syntonic symptoms pull the family together and are involved in the family structure through balance bargains.

If behaviors are completely syntonic, the family does not experience them as symptoms at all! It is not uncommon, for example, to see a youngster at the request of the school or court, only to learn that his symptomatic behaviors are highly syntonic to the family, which does not regard them as symptoms at all. In fact, the family often views the school or court as highly symptomatic!

Strictly speaking, the term syntonic symptom is contradictory unless there is a disparity of perception, as illustrated in the above example. Usually, of course, the overall picture involves sizable syntonic and dystonic elements. Families usually request removal of the dystonic elements and assume that they will be able to retain the syntonic elements. Therapy with families, as with individuals, may consist largely of elucidating the link between the two types of symptoms, and clinical resistance occurs when the family or patient is weighing the alternatives.

In summary, functioning requires that dystonic symptoms, which represent a reaction to severe and chronic stress, must become syntonic to the greatest extent possible. The alternative is to ignore the stress or attempt continuously to counteract it. The first alternative is dangerous; the second is expensive.

DEVELOPMENT AND MAINTENANCE OF SYMPTOMS

The easiest way to begin a discussion of how a family develops and maintains symptoms is to describe a situation where the symptoms have always been dystonic for a family. In an extreme case—tragically, a common one—the child's very existence has been dystonic to the family from the moment he was conceived. For example, a woman who discovers, after a tumultuous separation from her husband, that she is pregnant may hate the child months before it is born. Another family may reject a child because of its sex. In either situation, the extruded child presents an enormous clinical problem. Attempts to reintegrate (or, more accurately, integrate) him into his family are usually unsuccessful and are often accompanied by chaos, as illustrated in the following case:

> Bobbie, a clumsy and generally unlikely seven-year-old, was brought to the clinic by his parents, who complained about his periodic, unmanageable outbursts of temper. Because the parents believed that Bobbie would spend most of his life in a state hospital anyway, they regarded their request that we send him there forthwith as a reasonable one. During many months of therapy, this youngster enacted, through the use of dolls and the playhouse, the drama of the outsider who struggles to become an insider. Inevitably, his play revealed the outsider's violent rejection by those inside. On the few occasions when the outsider entered the house, a violent storm shook it, scattering its contents throughout the room. This scene was subsequently enacted by the family.
>
> During the final months of therapy, Bobbie was in fact integrated into his family. His grades improved dramatically, as did his peer relationships. At this point, his older brother,

who had seemed to be the most adaptive member of the family, stole a car and ran away from home. The family fell into a state of pandemonium. We speculate that previously established balance bargains had resulted in a rule that one member of the family would be outside. Therapy for the identified patient did not change this rule.

In many families, dystonic symptoms emerge over a long period if the child and his family are unable to get along smoothly. Any event may cause a variety of feelings, depending on whether it is experienced as facilitating or inhibiting adaptation (French & Steward, 1975). The same is true of parenting. Under optimal conditions, the child-parent system allows both members of each dyad to experience the joy of adaptive growth that occurs as they interact. The feedback processes are complex enough, however, so that innumerable factors may disrupt the interaction and generate bad feelings. A vicious spiral then occurs as depression and loss of self-esteem afflict the family. Any factor, such as a prolonged illness, that overtaxes the parents' ability to maintain their balance must be experienced as a stress. Children are a unique source of stress because they cannot easily be ignored or permanently avoided, although some families resort to these extreme measures. In this situation, the family is struggling with stress overload. The sequence is as follows: (1) stress arises as the family experiences difficulty caring for the child, (2) the child and family progressively experience more depression as their interactions become less and less gratifying, (3) complex processes establish the roles of bad child, angry mother, and so on, and (4) the family may seek help or resort to balance bargains or extrusion. Almost invariably, parents in this situation report: "We really *love* him, Doctor, we really do; but. . . . Well, to tell the truth, we don't *like* him."

The child's temperament is a particularly important source of difficulty. A mismatch between a child and his family can easily occur, creating the kind of stress overload described earlier. For example, if a woman who has always been meticulous about her own behavior, her house, and so forth delivers a child who is extremely active, has a short attention span, and reacts intensely, even to mild stimuli, it would be difficult for the two to generate a viable parent-child system. In other words, there would be a mismatch between the child's usual behavior and the expectations of his environment. Therefore, most of his behavior would place stress on the family and be labeled symptomatic, virtually from the outset, perhaps even before mother and child leave the hospital. In a different family, the same child might do well. An extended family that values physical activity and has many caretakers to deal with a challenging child might enjoy him. A placid child, on the other hand, would be considered optimal in the first environment and symptomatic in the second.

Again, it is important to emphasize the *symmetry* of this initial statement of imbalance. When we say that a child's temperament causes an imbalance within the family, we must be careful not to scapegoat the child! To do so would imply an overly simplified concept of the causality of symptoms and would amount to a demonology, with the family as a reference system and the child's temperament as the demon. The important point is that there is a *mismatch* between what the child's development requires and what the family is capable of providing.

The second major category of symptoms includes those that are partially syntonic—i.e., those that pull the family together and reduce its expenditure of energy and yet are disruptive to some degree. These symptoms are much more complex, evolve over a long period, and involve many levels of family functioning. Most of the literature published over the past 20 years has focused on symptoms that are partially syntonic (e.g., Framo, 1970; Mendell & Fisher, 1956; Satir, 1971). This type of behavior is usually operating when a family *voluntarily* brings a child in for professional evaluation and treatment but clings to the very symptoms that it finds distressing. To cope with the situation, the clinician must understand how the symptoms evolved. There are several possibilities.

First, the symptoms may have been syntonic for some family members and dystonic to others from the outset. If so, the clinician can infer that some family members are out of alignment with each other and that the child's behavior is supported by one parent, while viewed as symptomatic by the other. For example, a father who wants an active, vigorous child may be unhappy with a placid child, while his wife is pleased about the child's low level of activity. Thus there is disagreement within the family about what constitutes a symptom. This situation is obviously conducive to a serious power struggle related to a fundamental disagreement about the definition of acceptable behavior. The power struggle in this case involves not only the specific content of the child's behavior but the process of deciding who will determine how the family rules will be written.

A far more complex process involves the transition from a dystonic symptom to a syntonic symptom. It is here that the concept of the family as a system has its greatest power. The family proceeds along the lines already outlined: an imbalance within the system is dealt with by a balance bargain, which becomes irreversible, and a disease develops. On the political level, this process can be compared to the temporary delegation of extraordinary power to the leader of a country during a crisis. However, as Shakespeare beautifully illustrated in *The Tempest*, the tragic lesson of history is that this delegation of power tends to be irreversible, and the result is inexorable movement toward less diversity and flexibility in the governmental structure.

The loss of reversibility in this process is crucial. Consider a couple who, because of a severe emotional crisis, were unable to nurture their child adequately. When the child made reasonable demands for attention and affection, the parents were simply too exhausted to meet them and used food and toys as a substitute for attention. The child became a demanding brat, and the family encountered severe difficulty when it tried to reverse the pattern. (This phenomenon, called family turnover, will be discussed extensively in Chapter 8. See also Barcai & Rosenthal, 1974.)

A more complicated process is involved when the family has a fairly specific need for the child to assume a specific role within the family. The variety of roles that families require is enormous. Thus any personality pattern, no matter how pleasant or unpleasant or adaptive or maladaptive, may have developed in part because the family needed to have someone function in a particular way. We have already discussed the importance of the balance bargain in the development of symptoms, and the parameter of specificity might easily be included within this general concept. Every child is born with a sex, a specific temperament, and other characteristics. Every family at the time of a child's birth has created an enormously complex set of beliefs and wishes about what the child will do in and for the family. Ideally, of course, the family is prepared to offer a maximally adaptive environment for a child of either sex, any set of physical characteristics, and any temperament. But simple reality, not to mention the properties of the dynamic unconscious, precludes this possibility; there is no such thing as a perfect match between organism and environment. For example, we all have a complex structure of beliefs about what we will gain in a particular job, by driving a particular kind of car, by living in a particular neighborhood, by dressing a particular way; and so on. Similarly, certain intrinsic, biologically based characteristics in a child, such as sex, temperament, or appearance, will inevitably make it easy in some cases for parents to involve him in a balance bargain of some kind. It would be impossible—inappropriate in fact—for any organism to turn down such an opportunity. In essence, it amounts to the promise of a free lunch in violation of Commoner's fourth rule. In other words, the parents view the situation as a glorious opportunity to achieve two objectives at once: correct the imbalance they are struggling with on the one hand, and relate appropriately to the child on the other. Furthermore, the complexity of human behavior enables the family system to reinforce the behaviors that facilitate the necessary balance and avoid reinforcing those that will disrupt it. In adaptational terms, this maneuver may hold the promise that a Type II change is unnecessary—that the parents need not endure the painful and difficult process of change if only other family members will support their belief structure. Somehow, the special child makes it possible for the family to maintain balance, however poorly, by means of Type I processes alone. That is, the special child compensates for the family's inability to change, and we can confidently predict that efforts to alleviate the child's symptoms may meet with tremendous resistance!

It is never necessary to assume that the parent actively dislikes the child or actively plans to enmesh him in a hopeless tangle of role confusion, scapegoating, and the like. Parents and families, like all adaptive organisms, simply seek to reduce their expenditure of energy as efficiently as possible. For instance, consider Mr. and Mrs. J, whose families of origin were heavily enmeshed in the Game of Alcoholism (Berne, 1964). The model of close interpersonal relationships that both partners learned requires the role of Sickie (the alcoholic) and Wellie (the overcompensating partner who periodically rescues the alcoholic). In other words, both Mr. and Mrs. J are most familiar with relationships in which intimacy is expressed through the processes of illness and rescue. Thus they play some form of the Game of Alcoholism in most or all of their relationships. If the Js have a weak and sickly child with several congenital defects, they will be forced to spend an inordinate amount of time visiting physicians' offices, finding special schools for the child, and so forth. Acting adaptively, they will seize on the child's illnesses to accomplish two things simultaneously: satisfy their need to rescue the weak and express their loyalty to the familiar patterns of their families of origin. It will be impossible to see the maladaptive aspect of this family's rules until the family encounters a crisis. As predicted on the basis of the family history, the crisis occurred when the child became progressively less sick and more well and was eligible to attend a Boy Scout camp for normal rather than handicapped children. At this point, the family became chaotic; one result was no trip to the Scout camp for the child. The Js' maladaptive response to his improvement revealed the presence of the deeply buried balance bargain.

In Piagetian terms (which have the distinct advantage of being nonjudgmental as well as clear), we could say that the Js had previously constructed schemata for this situation. The set of stimuli associated with the Game of Alcoholism constituted aliment appropriate to these schemata. A change to different schemata would involve accommodation (or a Type II process), which is slow and sometimes painful. In learning-theory terms, we could state that the Js' early experiences had massively reinforced these behavior patterns. In any case, Mr. and Mrs. J are struggling with the universal issue of trying to maximize homeostasis while minimizing their expenditure of energy.

In summary, the family is an integrated system that functions according to a specific but often unconscious belief structure or mythology, which provides the reference norms or roles with respect to which the family functions. In addition to the role content, there is a specific set of rules for correcting deviations from reference norms (Type I processes) that also reveal the family's ability to shift its reference norms (Type II processes). The experience of intimacy requires that each family member recognize and follow the family's reference system. Therefore, conflict occurs if an individual's role is incompatible with his own adaptive strivings. A symptom always means that intrapsychic or interpersonal conflict exists somewhere in the system. Furthermore, a symptom can reflect a wide variety of fundamentally different phenomena. It can be dystonic—that is, it tends to push the family apart and increase the energy required to function, as in the case of a transient stress reaction. Or it can be syntonic—it tends to pull the family together and reduce the energy required to function, as in the case of symptomatic behaviors that have evolved gradually and are, by the time the family presents itself for clinical evaluation, deeply imbedded in the overall family processes. It is the second type of case that occupies most of the clinician's attention.

The systems concept implies that we need not, and in fact *cannot* scapegoat the family to explain syntonic symptoms. Family-syntonic symptoms are fundamentally adaptive maneuvers that have gone awry because they have become irreversible. Crises reveal the presence of these unwieldly, cumbersome, and maladaptive balance bargains. Yet crises also provide the system with an opportunity to rearrange itself into a more adaptive configuration. Thus the symptoms may cease, spontaneously or in response to treatment, and the entire family may improve.

In this chapter (adhering to the ancient tradition that physicians should focus on the morbid), I have emphasized the situation where the family becomes worse as the symptom-carrier improves. But it need not necessarily be so. The relationship of symptoms to the family structure is complex, and a shift in balance may move in one of several directions. In subsequent pages, I will offer some ideas for assessing whether a family is likely to improve or become worse.

No matter how hard we try to avoid it, there is always the danger that if we describe balance bargains, we will be viewed as accusatory or as resorting to an archaic disease model or medical model. As clinicians, we tend to be preoccupied with the unhealthy and lose sight of the fundamentally healthy, adaptive, striving nature of organisms. The distinction between health and pathology does not lie in any specific configuration of the system; it lies in the system's capacity to modify its configuration adaptively in response to the stresses or opportunities it encounters. It is human nature to seek continuously to violate the systems law that there is no free lunch and to be profoundly disappointed when we find that this law applies in every case! Life itself is fundamentally unbalanced. We are constantly changing open systems, attempting to make our way through a complex and occasionally difficult odyssey of life with a minimal expenditure of energy and minimal restructuring of our essential selves. These basic considerations may help us to understand that deeply human and tragic phenomenon, the family-syntonic symptom.

NOTES

*1. For a fascinating discussion of the changes in theoretical physics and their general implications, see Capek's remarkably readable book *The Philosophical Impact of Comtemporary Physics.*

Chapter 2

BASIC CLINICAL TOOLS AND THEIR USE

Chapter 1 outlined the fundamental concept of the system and defined a number of important terms, such as assimilation, accommodation, adaptation, Type I and Type II processes, and family belief structure. We attempted to apply these concepts to the mysterious fact that basically healthy, caring families develop serious problems, which, although painful and destructive, are nevertheless useful to them.

This chapter contains an evaluative outline that is useful in work with families and provides the structure for Chapters 3 through 7. But before presenting the outline, I will review several additional concepts that appear throughout the book. The first section discusses five important clinical tools: (1) temperamental type, (2) the concept of epigenesis, (3) affect, (4) problem-solving styles, and (5) degree of differentiation. The second section, titled "Data Collection and Case Formulation," contains my own views about the challenge of the data-collection process and the limitations and implications of psychiatric labels.

Major Clinical Tools

Temperamental Type

The work of Thomas, Chess, and Birch (1970) on differences in temperament is essential reading for anyone who works with families and children. The concept of behavioral individuality in infancy is based on the following facts: (1) brain structure, like all other biological phenomena, varies from one individual to another (i.e., we all look different on the outside and we are all wired differently on the inside), (2) brain structure relates to behavior, and therefore (3) temperament, the biological anlage of personality, is also unique. In other words, each child is born with a specific temperamental type, which Thomas and his colleagues define as the set of behavioral and response patterns that are uniquely his own.

Temperamental type can be divided into nine different traits: level of activity, rhythmicity, approach/withdrawal, adaptability, intensity of reaction, quality of mood, persistence/attention span, distractibility, and reaction threshold. Because each trait varies independently, an incredibly wide variety of temperaments is possible. For example, taking only the extremes of each trait would give us a total of 2^9, or 512 different temperaments. The following list of the nine traits contains a brief description of typical behavior at each end of the spectrum:

Activity Level. Is the child constantly on the move, or does he tend to be passive physically?

Rhythmicity. Does he eat, sleep, and have bowel movements according to a relatively predictable schedule, or does he carry out these functions on a seemingly random basis?

Approach/withdrawal. Does the child tend to approach new situations willingly, or does he tend to hang back?

Adaptability. Does he tolerate change and respond easily to suggestions or discipline, or do these events disturb him?

Intensity of reaction. Does he react intensely to emotional situations, both positive and negative, or does he tend to be somewhat bland?

Quality of mood. Is he usually cheerful, or does he tend to be negative and ornery?

Persistence/attention span. Does he devote his attention to one thing for long periods, or does he turn his attention to something else relatively quickly?

Distractibility. Is he easily distracted, or does he tend to persist in what he is doing despite distractions?

Reaction threshold. Is he a "hair-trigger kid," i.e., does he react even to mild stimuli, or does it take a strong stimulus to set him off?

Table 2.1   Three General Temperamental Types

Type	Traits					
	Activity level	Rhythmicity	Approach/ withdrawal	Adapt- ability	Intensity of reaction	Quality of mood
Easy	Variable	High	Approach	High	Low	Positive
Slow to warm up	Low or moderate	Variable	Initial withdrawal	Slow	Moderate	Slightly negative
Difficult	Variable	Low	Withdrawal	Slow	High	Negative

Source: Thomas, Chess & Birch, 1970.

In practice, these traits tend to cluster into three relatively distinct temperamental types: "easy," "slow to warm up," and "difficult." Table 2.1 illustrates these three general types, based on the first six traits, which Thomas and his colleagues found were sufficient to establish a child's overall temperament.

Epigenetic Development

Workers in a variety of fields, including embryology (Waddington, 1962), cognitive development (Piaget, 1970), psychosocial development (Erikson, 1950) have contributed to the resolution of the nature-nurture controversy. The term epigenetic summarizes their position on this critical issue. We must account for both biological factors and environmental-interactional factors. In discussing Waddington's use of the term epigenetic, Piaget stated that

> the main characteristics of . . . epigenetic development are not only the well-known and obvious ones of succession in sequential order and of progressive integration . . . but also some less obvious ones. . . . [which act] in such a way that if an external influence causes the developing organism to deviate from . . . [a developmental sequence, the organism reacts in a way that] tends to channel it back to the normal sequence or, if this fails, switches it to a new . . . [sequence] as similar as possible to the original one [1970, p. 710].

On the biological level, the embryologist must explain the organism's final form as the result of the interaction between the basic information available to the organism in its genetic material, the limitations and capabilities of the other parts of its cells, and the environment.

In coping with the same problem in the area of cognitive development, Piaget (1970, 1972) arrived at the same concept, which he called interactional structuralism: i.e., interaction between the organism's unique potential and the environment's unique characteristics creates a unique set of cognitive structures. Erikson (1950) also used the epigenetic concept in his work on psychosexual and psychosocial development. He has been concerned with the specific individual, cultural, and family characteristics that interact to generate a unique personality. Thus the epigenetic concept has been enormously useful at the biological, cognitive, and psychosocial levels.

Here, I have organized the topic of cognitive and psychosocial-psychosexual development around Piaget's concepts of preoperational and operational thought (Flavell, 1963) and Erikson's "The Eight Ages of Man" (1950).

COGNITIVE DEVELOPMENT.   According to Piaget, there is a critical difference between preoperational logic of the child and the operational logic of the adult. In his summary of the cognitive processes of preschool children, Flavell (1963) lists the following as the primary characteristics of preoperational thought: (1) egocentrism, the tendency to assume that the self is the focus of events, (2) magical causality, which permits the child to assume a causal relationship between events on the basis of highly idiosyncratic associations, (3) centration, the inability to subdivide a complex field of events into independently variable components, and (4) the tendency to handle problems by action and to focus on states rather than on the possibility of transformation. In other words, the child is forced to generalize in a way that in an adult would be characterized immediately as neurotic thought: e.g., "I played with my dog and got sick and had to be in isolation, and the dog was put to sleep forever. Therefore, I am dangerous."

In contrast, operational thought is characterized by the ability to use reversible internal representations of external acts and by the recognition that these internal representations can be moved about, in thought, with complete reversibility—which is a far more efficient way to proceed than is testing out each possibility operationally. Thus the operational thinker is able to scan a large number of options in a situation and choose the most suitable one.

The magical causality and egocentrism that characterize preoperational thought cannot be overemphasized. Some of the greatest cognitive challenges that an individual must deal with throughout his entire life are encountered during the preoperational stage, when only a primitive, qualitative kind of logic is available. Consider, for example, the fact that people come in *two different kinds*—a mind-boggling fact if ever there was one! How is the young mind to explain it? Similarly, the vicissitudes of the family triangle, or Oedipal complex, must be handled with preoperational logic. Is it any wonder that the child's solutions to these enormous problems lead to fantasy structures that seem bizarre when observed retrospectively during the psychoanalysis of an adult!

Preoperational logic accounts for the "cute" nature of children's descriptions of the world. The Winnie the Pooh Stories contain numerous examples. For instance, Pooh grasps a balloon and ascends into the air, stopping when he reaches the bees and their honey. In other words, the physics of Pooh's universe operate with respect to his interest in honey, and we would expect Pooh's explanation of this phenomenon to include both egocentrism and magical causality.

PSYCHOSOCIAL-PSYCHOSEXUAL DEVELOPMENT.   I have chosen to organize this section around Erik Erikson's work, particularly his essay "The Eight Ages of Man," published in *Childhood and Society*. The first five stages of development are summarized in Table 2.2.

Erikson has generalized Sigmund Freud's work in the area of psychosexual development in a way that makes it easier to understand and use. But how exactly does his thinking differ from Freud's? Perhaps Freud's concept of fixation point best illustrates the contrast. In discussing the salmon-fishing culture of Native Americans in the northwestern United States, Erikson noted that hoarding salmon over a period of months was necessary for survival in that environment. The tribes ability to mold the child's development in a way that increases this hoarding tendency could be viewed in Freudian terms as facilitating an anal fixation in psychosexual development. In Erikson's view, it

Table 2.2 A Summary of Erikson's First Five Ages of Man

Stage	Corresponding Freudian phase	Opportunities	Dangers	Optimal outcome
I. Basic trust vs. mistrust	Infancy (oral phase)	I experience the environment as nurturing, reliable, and trustworthy. I am cared for.	I have been abandoned.	Capacity for intimacy.
II. Autonomy vs. shame and doubt	Toddlerhood (anal phase)	I own and like my body, and I am in control of myself and my bodily functions.	My body and I are bad. Therefore, I must carefully control everything I do.	Self-control without loss of self-esteem. Appropriate love-hate ratio.
III. Initiative vs. guilt	Preschool (phallic phase)	I can do lots of exciting things. Sometimes my powers seem almost magical!	Sometimes I am terrified that others will be so angry at me for what I want to do that they will harm or destroy me.	Simultaneous access to and appropriate control of impulses.
IV. Industry vs. inferiority	Elementary School (latency phase)	I enjoy doing and achieving because it gives me satisfaction, recognition from others, and good opportunities to relate to other people.	I am worthless. At best, I can only achieve (worthless) recognition for things I do or produce.	Sufficient extension of ego boundaries so that self-esteem can be gained through achievement.

| V. Identity vs. role confusion | Adolescence | I know who I am, and I want to make this distinct, unique self apparent both to myself and the world as I create my adult life. | I have no idea who I am or where I am going. | A good sense of personal identity and the capacity to relate to the world in terms of this identity. |

Source: Erikson, 1950.

would represent the necessary "fine tuning" of the relationship between the individual and his environment. The fact that a developing personality can take on a wide variety of configurations is part of the beauty and adaptiveness of humanity. Removed from its initial context, however, a personality may be maladaptive; hence we make the value judgment implicit in the term personality disorder.

If we discuss the structure of the personality in psychosexual terms, a simple fixation point that is clearly related to a specific developmental event (or trauma) and to a specific cluster of symptoms, would be a rare event indeed. The development of a unique personality is always adaptive in some context. As Nagera stated:

> It is important to re-emphasize that the impact of developmental interferences on the child's future development varies greatly with the age of the child, the level of ego and drive development at the time of the interference, as well as with other factors. While not all developmental interferences automatically damage the structure of the personality, there can be little doubt that many personalities are decisively shaped by such interferences, especially if they occur at crucial developmental phases and are operative for a prolonged period of time [1966, p. 37]."

Why is Erikson's concept of psychosexual stages valuable? Its value lies in its ability to help us translate from

clinical observation to underlying feelings and back to predictions about behavior. The different stages are described
in terms that are general enough to render them virtually
culture free: they are the organizing opportunity-disaster
pairs that characterize a series of developmental plateaus.

For example, Stage I (infancy) presents the child with
an opportunity to develop basic trust: "Will my average
expectable behavior interact with the average expectable
environment in such a way that homeostasis is maintained?" The development of the infant-caretaker system is
influenced by innumerable factors on many levels. Basic
mistrust is the disastrous outcome of this stage of development: "I can assume that the average expectable interaction between myself and the environment will go badly for
me."

In Stage II (toddlerhood) the child has the opportunity
to develop autonomy: "I have good control of my body and
its relationship to the environment. I am in love with the
world, which I can explore." The complexity of developing
the full potential of a stage while retaining the best of the
prior stage is, of course, first encountered during the transition between Stage I and Stage II. "If I develop autonomy, must I give up the warmth and intimacy of Stage I?
Can I have both?" The disaster of Stage II is a sense of
shame and a sense of doubt about one's worth.

Stage III (latency) is interesting because the impact of
the Freudian concept of the Oedipal complex has been so
great. Newly endowed with "free possession of a surplus of
energy which permits him to forget failures quickly and to
approach what seems desirable. . . . [Erikson, 1950, p. 235]-
", the child is faced with wonderful new opportunities. But
using his surplus of free energy in the wrong direction may
lead to guilt. The opportunity to develop initiative is thus
counterbalanced by the disaster of overwhelming guilt.

Note the disappearance of the argument between the
psychoanalytic point of view that the Oedipal complex is

the core of psychosexual development and the view of some anthropologists that the absence of an Oedipal triangle in some cultures disproves the psychoanalytic point of view. If the opportunity of healthy initiative and the disaster of excessive guilt are the organizing forces around which development occurs, the specific content of the child's experience is irrelevant. One may take the initiative toward any object and experience guilt about having done so; the object need not necessarily be the parent of the opposite sex.)

A good understanding of these three developmental stages will advance clinical work a long way. If your goal is an increased ability to empathize with your patients, read Erikson's "The Eight Ages of Man" many times and translate your raw clinical data into the terms he provides.

The concept of temperamental type complements Erikson's developmental stages beautifully, for a child's temperament clearly has a critical bearing on how the child will cope with the developmental tasks that are specific to each stage. For example, rhythmicity may be crucially important during Stage I; distractibility and persistence/attention span may be critical during Stage II, and so on.

Translating the concept of epigenesis into an appropriate method of interviewing is not easy. I strongly urge you to obtain from any source available a conceptualization of the major developmental events of each stage and to become facile in its clinical application.

Affect

Although affect is a concept dear to the heart of psychiatric clinicians, a clear and clinically useful definition is difficult to find. Affect can be defined as a set of qualitatively specific signals that inform the organism about the survival value of a particular situation or course of action. Therefore, we frequently ask patients "How do you feel about that?" because it is an appropriate way to find out an individual's estimate of the probability that a situation or course of action has good survival value for him. From a systems perspective, French and Steward (1975) have described the heuristic value of a model that proposes a pair of primary affects associated with Type I processes, or assimilation (anxiety and pleasure), and another pair associated with Type II processes, or accommodation (grief and satisfaction). This results in four primary affects and four secondary affects (joy, greed, depression, and guilt), which are combinations of the primary ones. The advantage of this scheme is that affect can be defined in general terms. It is therefore appropriate to talk about depression in children, although the word depression was, until recently, conspicuously absent from the literature in child psychiatry.

Affect, then, is a general term for a set of signals about how things are going. Mood, or the predominant affect over a period of time, like all other behaviors, is the result of the interaction between biological and interactional factors.

Earlier, I discussed the intrinsic biological component of mood as a temperamental trait. Here we will consider the final result. To the extent that mood reflects experience, it can be conceptualized as the child's overall estimate of the probability that a randomly selected encounter between the self and the environment will have a good outcome. In children, as in adults, affect should be variable and appropriate to content. Health or pathology lies in the appropriateness of the response to the current realities of life, and the distinction between a *reversible,* appropriate stress reaction and a fixed depressive mood is crucial.

The concept of depression in children bears further discussion. A major event in child psychiatry was the publication in 1971 of Malmquist's article on depression in children and adolescents, which extended Glaser's finding (1967) that depression in children and adolescents takes a variety of forms and proposed a comprehensive classification. In 1972 Cytryn and McKnew suggested a simpler, more clinically useful classification: children can express depression through anxiety, withdrawal, or hostility. In my opinion, depression may be the most commonly misdiagnosed condition in child psychiatry as well as in internal medicine. This is especially true when a child does not appear to be sad. The issue in depression is not sadness but a sense of hopelessness and helplessness (Engel, 1968). A child can express these feelings about his relationship to the world by acting-out behaviors or by passive withdrawal.

In summary, affect is the set of signals that indicates how well an individual's adaptive processes are functioning. Fixed affect indicates internal distress of some sort. If depression is defined in sufficiently general terms, the concept can be applied to children.

Problem-Solving Style

The problem-solving style of any system can be determined by examining how the system functions during a crisis. A crisis generates an unusual configuration from which otherwise unavailable and unique information can be extracted. For instance, a parent may say: "I never really knew how much I cared about my son until he was so sick," or "I always knew that my job was important to me, and I kind of assumed that my family would always be there. I never realized how important my family was to me until my wife began talking about splitting up."

Although clinical data can be organized according to many conceptual models, most clinicians use some form of the concept of the psychosexual development discussed earlier. In general, any organism in any situation must estimate the probability that a certain course of action will maximize homeostasis and minimize the need for accommodation. In other words, we are constantly challenged to seek the most adaptive course of action. The concept of psychosexual stages can be linked to this general concept of organism function.

PSYCHOSEXUAL STAGE AND AFFECT.   Consider Erikson's conceptualization that all children, regardless of culture, must deal with issues of basic trust versus basic mistrust during infancy, with the issue of misuse of autonomy versus shame and doubt during toddlerhood, and so on. Now consider the adult who must decide which course of action will be most adaptive in a particular situation. One key aspect of the problem is that he must decide "which aspect of adaptation is currently the most important to me? Should I focus my energy primarily upon keeping myself fed and sheltered? Should I focus on the need to function as an individual despite my need for interpersonal relationships? Do I have the realities of life sufficiently well in hand so that I can afford the luxury of a creative artistic endeavor?" The ideally adaptive individual would scan all possible alternatives and make the best possible decision in each instance. But real people are not ideally adaptive!

The term fixation neatly summarizes this complex developmental-behavioral viewpoint. An individual may, as a function of previous experience, assign an inordinately high significance, in a randomly selected situation, to issues that are relevent to earlier developmental levels. Thus it is clinically useful to make two assumptions: (1) previous experience influences the kind of probability estimates that an adult will make about the most adaptive course of action and (2) there is a qualitative specificity to learning at each psychosexual stage. Obviously, the same conclusions could be reached from a wide variety of theoretical viewpoints. In short, it is useful to ask: Are this individual's estimates about the adaptive value of a particular course of action biased unduly by concerns that characterize a particular developmental stage? For example, is he prone to evaluate the trust-mistrust aspects of the problem, or does he focus too much attention on the aspects of autonomy versus shame and doubt?

Clinically, one gains leverage on this problem by observing not only the predominant themes a patient presents but also his feeling tone. Feelings are a set of qualitatively specific signals that inform the organism about the advisability of pursuing or abandoning a particular course of action. In other words, our feelings tell us what our probability estimate is about the adaptiveness of a certain course of action. In general, we assume clinically that psychosexual stages have fairly characteristic feeling tones: e.g., warmth versus loneliness (Stage I), the excited pride of autonomy versus shame and doubt (Stage II), the eager excitement of initiative versus guilt (Stage III), the joy of creative industry versus inferiority (Stage IV), and so on.

CLINICAL CONSIDERATIONS.   Returning to the clinical problem of speaking to the parents of a child in trouble, let us attempt to cull some clinical leverage from these concepts. If a family's problem-solving style is flexible and adaptive in a variety of situations, if their feeling tone is variable and content-appropriate, if family members speak in fairly random sequence, and if the child's symptoms do not seem to be syntonic for the entire family, then the clinician is fairly safe in assuming that vigorous pursuit of a predominate influence from any one of the psychosexual levels will not be rewarding.

The reverse would be true, of course, in a rigid and maladaptive family. If a couple function in a manner that is consistent with a particular psychosexual level and if there is a high degree of reliability in this regard from one situation to the next (for example, tone of voice during an intake phone call, the nature of the presenting problem, the couple's behavior in the waiting room and during sessions, the clinician can begin to construct the working hypothesis that this couple will approach all life problems assuming that the significant issues are those of a particular psychosexual stage. For example, if the clinician hears a whining, frightened voice during an initial telephone call, sees an eight-year-old child leaning on an obese mother in the waiting room, and obtains a family history of alcoholism and a chief complaint of school phobia, he is entitled to begin constructing the working hypothesis that this family system tends to approach life with the attitude that issues of trust and mistrust are paramount. If this is so, there will be important implications for treatment.

First, buried somewhere in the family, there is likely to be a large bolus of feelings connected with abandonment and loss, and much of the family distortion may be related to one members attempts to protect himself against these painful feelings. In other words, a family member in a position of power may have "wrapped" the family around his own feelings as a protective covering. Therefore, if a family chronically assumes the configuration that is characteristic of a stressed family, even in the absence of a visible source of stress, it may be responding to the source of stress within one person.

Second, if this is the case, it follows that the family can return to a more nearly normal configuration if the person in power learns to deal with these feelings more appropriately.

Third, the therapist will be forewarned about the type of issues in which he will eventually become involved. For instance, is the family likely to resent his vacations and other absences (Stage I)? Are there likely to be power struggles (Stage II)? Is competition between the therapist and family members likely to occur (Stage III)?

Fourth, if the therapist has reason to believe that the identified patient's symptoms are directly related to the conflict experienced by the person in power, it may be appropriate to help him express this conflict appropriately in the playroom.

The concept of psychosexual stages helps the clinician to draw inferences about a patient's underlying feelings. It is similar to the mathematical tools that the seismographer uses to measure surface vibrations and draw inferences about deep structures. An understanding of underlying affect is essential to empathy. Erikson's general formulation concerning the conflicts that occur at each developmental stage is more useful to most clinicians than is the classical Freudian concept of fixation points.

Degree of Differentiation

Degree of differentiation (Bowen, 1966) can be defined in a variety of ways. First, we can view it as the probability that an individual will select a problem-solving maneuver from among those provided by his family. In other words, it represents the nuclear family's library of problem-solving maneuvers. The individual with a low degree of differentiation will inevitably handle all problems by using one of the solutions already worked out by his family. Indeed, he must do so because if he chooses another coping maneuver, his family is likely to view this as a serious break with the core belief structure. A more highly differentiated individual not only has access to the family library but is free to create new solutions without being penalized by the family.

Another way to look at the degree of differentiation is in terms of the density of the social field. Density does not mean the number of people who occupy the field; it means the force with which the social field influences our reference individual. Because the structure of the poorly differentiated family exerts an enormous influence, family members tend to orbit around the family much as a moon orbits around a planet; the motion of the moon can be predicted, based on the simple physical parameters of the system. Its orbit can change only when there is a cataclysmic event of some kind, such as the entry into the gravitational field of a second mass large enough to compete successfully with the first.

ADAPTABILITY.   The concept of differentiation neatly coincides with that of role rigidity versus role flexibility. A poorly differentiated family does not permit individual members to deviate from prescribed roles. A highly differentiated family, on the other hand, not only permits but encourages self-definition of roles. Role rigidity and differentiation can also be viewed according to the rules of adaptation, especially those pertaining to Type II processes. The rules of adaptation in a poorly differentiated family do not provide for a shift in belief structure: i.e., a poorly differentiated, role-rigid family cannot make Type II changes. Therefore, one of its rules of adaptation is: "No major shifts in belief structure will occur in this family," or "We believe that if any major shift in our belief structure occurs, the results will be disastrous."

INTROJECTION AND PSYCHOSEXUAL STAGE.   The degree of differentiation is also compatible with two important psychoanalytic concepts: introjection and psychosexual development. The introject is the internal representation of the parent. If the introject is extremely rigid and if the individual is bound by the introject's demands, that individual will not deviate much from the family pattern.

The following discussion about the different levels of differentiation corresponds well with the earlier discussions about psychosexual stages, problem-solving style, and epigenetic development. Poorly differentiated families are described in terms that are similar to those used to describe an individual who approaches life's problems assuming that Stage I issues are of utmost importance. That is, family members tend to protect themselves against feelings of abandonment and isolation. Somewhat more differentiated families usually engage in power struggles when an individual member attempts to establish his autonomy from, yet is closely bound to the nuclear family. Members of families in the middle range of differentiation tend to move somewhat overconfidently into the world and periodically experience humiliating defeats. Members of highly differentiated families are similar to self-actualizing individuals: in other words, family members are simultaneously autonomous and capable of close sharing among themselves.

TEMPERAMENT AND COGNITIVE ABILITY.   In operational terms, a family's degree of differentiation is closely related to two other factors: the temperamental types of the children and the cognitive capacities of individual family members. One important question in child-family psychiatry concerns the fact that in a family of many children, one or two children may be selected as the sacrificial lambs while the others function well. A child's temperament may be a crucial factor here. Consider two children who are opposites in each of the following traits: mood, approach/withdrawal, and adaptability. The child who tends to handle novelty by withdrawal, exhibits a negative mood, and adapts to change with great difficulty will obviously be prone to stay close to home and therefore be at great risk for intrafamily influences. The child who responds to novelty with approach, is usually cheerful, and adapts readily to new situations will be able to move out of the nuclear family and explore other resources in the environment. Thus these three traits alone might readily explain the fact that two children (who for the sake of argument are otherwise identical) would be in radically different positions with respect to the risk that the nuclear family will require them to fill special roles which might be maladaptive for them as individuals.

Piaget's concept of preoperational thought (Flavell, 1963) is useful when discussing the second crucial factor— the cognitive capacities of individual family members. Let's look at the child's inability to subdivide the perceptual field into a number of components. Differentiation requires a certain capacity for decentration. If the individual can make only one judgment at a time about a complex conceptual field (e.g., "my parents" or "my family"), he must view the family as all good or all bad. The consequences of this are serious. If an individual must view his family as all good, he has no option but to accept its recommendations concerning his behavior. If he must view his family as all bad, he is forced to develop a poor self-image or grieve the loss of his entire family. The more highly differentiated individual can say: "Considering all the interactions between myself and my nuclear family, it is clear that some interactions are very good and have resulted in growth for all members concerned. On the other hand, other interactions have been expensive and bothersome for me as well as for others." This type of complex cognitive maneuver rests on the capacity to perform decentration.

The implications of egocentrism and magical thinking are also clear in this regard. If an individual sees himself as the center of the known universe and if events are causally linked to each other in a magical way, his attempts to differentiate himself from the nuclear family may be disastrous because he is held solely responsible.

Finally, because the preoperational child's inability to carry out reversible, internal representations of behaviors makes experimentation expensive, the child can determine the outcome of his behavior only by direct experimentation. He is unable to predict the sequence of events that might reasonably follow a certain action and to make a judgment based on his prediction. In summary, a primitive cognitive structure characterized by qualitative thinking of the preoperational type leaves the child with only one option—to maintain an extremely close, poorly differentiated relationship with his nuclear family.

Preoperational thought is normal in the preschool child. But clinicians will immediately recognize that some adults and families function in ways that are virtually identical to those of the preoperational child of a poorly differentiated family. In other words, neurotic adults function as though an inner voice were telling them: "If you deviate from this reference structure, an enormous irreversible disaster will immediately befall you."

THE FAMILY'S LEVEL OF DIFFERENTIATION.   The term differentiation creates a problem of nomenclature. Bowen (1966), for example, used the term differentiation and devised a scale ranging from 0 to 100, which he divided into quartiles. Hoover and Franz (1972) proposed the inverse concept of degree of entanglement and divided the range into five different levels. I prefer the term differentiation because of its more optimistic tone. But it seems more appropriate to talk about general levels of differentiation than to attempt precise estimates such as percentage differentiation. Thus degree of differentiation will be discussed in this book in terms of the following five levels (modified from Bowen, 1966, and Hoover & Franz, 1972):

Level 1. Families at this level contain one or more members who are virtually symbiotic with the entire family or with individual members. *Folie a deux* patterns and symbiotic psychoses are common. Although the overall family structure does not change, family members often play musical chairs with roles: e.g., if an alcoholic stops drinking, his spouse may begin drinking. When the family feels cornered, it will immediately terminate therapy and often will leave the area. To have a significant therapeutic experience, an individual from this type of family must grieve the loss of large segments of the family belief structure. Significant and prolonged depression is a virtual necessity during this process, and the end result of treatment is minimal interest in the family of origin.

Level 2. Family members either struggle actively to maintain a sense of autonomy by open rebellion or hostility or, at the other extreme, are overly dependent. They live close together or, if geographically separated, contact one another frequently; these contacts consume an enormous amount of their time and energy. Individuals are often engaged in hard versions of life games, such as alcoholism, which may be played to the point of severe illness or death. These families are characterized by strong alliances, strong barriers, repetition of maladaptive life-styles, and some members who are extremely symptomatic and at least one member who is seemingly above reproach. Alcoholism, gambling, excessive devotion to religion or a career—anything that serves a coercive interpersonal function—are common. Although significant structural, or Type II changes can occur, they are usually accompanied by severe turbulence. Suicidal threats, for example, are common during a crisis. The family often includes a person who has the privilege of avoiding Type II changes by manipulating others, and other family members usually protect, defend, and are tremendously loyal to him. Frequently, homeostasis is maintained through guilt: "I could never do anything that would hurt poor Mother (or any person who is privileged to avoid Type II changes).

Level 3. Although these families exhibit an adequate degree of autonomy in many areas, individual members may find that the prevailing family opinion is the deciding factor in their lives. A variety of family myths exist, and members often pay a high price in the form of pressure from other members for deviating significantly from these myths. Generally speaking, however, family members are able to live reasonably autonomous lives and maintain constructive contacts with one another. The ability of Level 3 families to make Type II changes varies in terms of probability and cost.

Level 4. Although members of Level 4 families achieve an adequate degree of autonomy, they periodically must isolate themselves to an extent to maintain balance. Some areas of function may be strongly influenced by the family belief structure, but serious entanglements seldom or never occur. Type I and II maneuvers are usually used appropriately.

Level 5. Members of Level 5 families live their own lives and consult one another when it is appropriate: i.e., they are in touch with but not ruled by the family. They accept the similarities and differences among family members, are both loving and autonomous, and can manage variations in interpersonal distance without difficulty. At the theoretical upper end of this level is the completely self-actualizing individual who can balance Type I and Type II processes.

A correct evaluation of a family's capacity to facilitate differentiation among its members is crucial. It is fair to say that no other clinical tool can save the clinician more grief. Conversely, if a clinician is having trouble with a case, it is a safe bet that he has overestimated the family's degree of differentiation.

Each of the clinical tools described in this section is analogous to an enormous iceberg—we have been able to survey only the uppermost surface. The good clinician has a variety of tools at his disposal and can apply them selectively and appropriately. But the five reviewed here, if used in concert appropriately, have enormous power.

DATA COLLECTION AND CASE FORMULATION

Before presenting the evaluative outline that provides the structure for most of this book, I want to discuss the general problem of making decisions and predictions in the face of uncertainty, particularly in medicine, and the specific problems raised by psychiatric diagnosis.[1]

The objective of an evaluation is the ability to predict, and we gather information for this reason alone. The evaluation must lead to recommendations for intervention. How do we proceed from data to diagnosis or formulation?

Data and Their Vicissitudes

The first thing we need is an adequate data base, but clinical observations are beset by an abysmally bad signal-to-noise ratio. Although a vast amount of news is available, little of it is data. The problem is to extract the useful information from the noise. The fable about a man who made a bargain with a troll illustrates this problem. The troll promised the man a pot of gold in return for his daughter; he would find the gold the following morning under a tree marked with the troll's red bandana. In the morning the man, having delivered his daughter to the troll, returned to the woods to find that all the trees were festooned with red bandanas. The troll had kept his promise, but had created a signal-to-noise ratio that made it impossible for the man to extract the essential information.

Clinically, we are in a similar position; the problem is not to find a signal, but a signal that means something. Fortunately, however, there are abundant opportunities to observate repetitive patterns. We can collect an enormous amount of data through a preliminary telephone call, and we gain additional critical information by observing a family as it walks into the clinic or sits in the waiting room. We obtain even more information as a family walks from the waiting room to the office; as members arrange themselves in the office; and as they communicate verbally, intraverbally and nonverbally with each other and with us.

The challenge in gathering data is to make as many separate observations as possible (Campbell & Stanley, 1963). We are tempted to make the minimum number of observations necessary for an initial impression and then bias our subsequent observations so that we "observe" what we expect. In so doing, however, we reduce the number of independent observations to an extremely small number.[2] The skillful clinician, faced with a diagnostic problem, continually sees the patient anew. Because labels tend to bias further perceptions, we should label late and reluctantly. Remember that outflow from the brain influences perception at the first synapse!

Having obtained a reasonable data base, how should we proceed? In general, data can be used in one of two ways: to exclude or support reasonable possibilities. The first use is by far the more powerful since a contradictory observation is both necessary and sufficient to exclude an hypothesis. Therefore, competent clinicians proceed by the well-known "rule-out" method. Psychiatrists are not as facile at doing so as other clinicians, however; too often, we proceed by considering data that support our diagnostic impressions.

Our clinical task is further complicated by the necessity of making a decision despite uncertainty. Physicians and patients have struggled with this problem in many ways, and the results often reflect the intensity of both the patients' and physicians' wish for diagnostic and therapeutic certainty rather than respect for the limitations of clinical judgment. In fact, the physician's historical role more closely resembles that of a shaman or medicine man than of a scientist. This priestly role sometimes overrides our respect for the limitations of our diagnostic skills. Although nonphysicians may be equally sloppy, the enormous social and legal importance of a psychiatric diagnosis, which often rests, fairly or unfairly (probably unfairly), on a simple medical model of psychological dysfunction, should make us especially cautious.

Kahneman and Tversky pointed out that "in making predictions and judgments under uncertainty . . . people predict by representativeness, that is, they select or order outcomes by the degree to which the outcomes represent the essential features of the evidence [1973, pp. 237–238]." In other words, we are prone to make predictions based on a comparison between the clinical picture as we see it, on the one hand, and our stereotypes of the class of disorders we associate with the clinical picture, on the other. This problem-solving process does not take into account the prevalence of different types of disorders in the general population. (Consequently, rare conditions such as early infantile autism tend to be overdiagnosed.) Furthermore, we usually lack the means to assess the reliability of our own clinical impressions and our stereotypes about the class of disorders we associate with the patient. Because we tend to have more confidence in predictions about extremely good or extremely poor performance (Johnson, 1972), we are likely to have more confidence in a grim diagnosis than in a benign one. Consider, for example, how traumatic a premature diagnosis of severe retardation, schizophrenia, or autism is for a family.

Other sources of errors in judgment can be paraphrased as follows (Kahneman & Tversky, 1973; Hoffman, & Slovik & Rorer, 1968): How many of us are prone to state grandly "In my clinical experience. . . ." when our sample consists of only a few cases? How often do we use a diagnosis as a permanent label rather than as a probability estimate? How often do we defend a clinical judgment by saying "Just last week I saw a case of . . ." or "I have seen enough cases like this to know that. . . .?" And how often do we fall in love with a clever diagnosis and ignore subsequent data that contradict it?

Clinicians sometimes defend themselves by maintaining that in fact they have considered not only a large number of parameters in making a clinical judgment but the interaction between important variables. This attractive argument, however, may not be valid. In a study of clinical judgment, Hoffman, Slovik, and Rorer stated that "the largest main *effect* usually accounted for 10 to 40 times as much of the total variance in the judgments as the largest *interaction* [1968, p. 343; italics added]." Thus the burden of proof is shifting. He who claims diagnostic certainty will be challenged to make explicit his data base, inferential processes, and level of confidence.

Diagnosis Versus Formulation

HAZARDS OF DIAGNOSIS.   In child and family psychiatry, the data are not only extremely complex but frequently unreliable because we must rely on the reports of teachers and parents and on time-limited and environmentally biased samples of information gathered in our own offices. Furthermore, there are enormous subjective biases. These can be observed at any staff conference where one clinician wants to "diagnose" the child, another wants to "diagnose" the parents, and a heated argument ensues. Finally, the fact that children are, by definition, growing and developing organisms raises serious questions about the feasibility of diagnosing children.

What is a diagnosis? Formally, a diagnosis is a statement that rests on classic Aristotelian logic. If we say that an individual falls within class X, we can safely conclude that he has all the characteristics of class X. Therefore, if we say that an individual is diabetic, we can infer that he exhibits all the characteristics of diabetes. This kind of cataloging statement has served physicians fairly well as an essential shorthand for rapid communication. Its limitations and dangers are inherent in the limitations of class-inclusion logic. A diagnosis is a description that pulls together an etiology (a cause), a pathogenesis (the sequence of processes whereby the cause leads to the disease), a syndrome (a collection of symptoms and signs characteristic of the illness), and typical treatment and clinical course. A formal diagnosis can be no more useful as a problem-solving tool than the classic Aristotelian logic on which it rests, and Aristotelian logic is, by its very nature, inadequate to account for the complex, multiply determined, continually shifting processes we encounter in psychiatry—and especially in child and family psychiatry. Furthermore, a diagnosis represents a negative bias because its purpose is to describe an individual's *least* adaptive aspects. In biological medicine, the negative bias is not dangerous; a diagnosis of congestive heart failure is a useful way for physicians to communicate to each other a host of information that is relevant to treatment. It is not used to label the patient as a no-goodnik. However, behavioral and psychiatric labels such as hyperactive or schizophrenic have a much greater splatter effect and tend to cast aspersions on the individual in a global way. Unfortunately, this hazard is forever present because of the tendency to draw inferences from labels, no matter how meticulous the clinician may have been. This is particularly tragic in child psychiatry because we are dealing with developing organisms.

POWER OF FORMULATION.   In contrast to a diagnosis, a formulation has a far greater descriptive and explanatory power. A formulation is to a general systems approach to illness what diagnosis is to the Aristotelian approach. A formulation can be defined as a description of an individual, family, or social system that includes a statement about each of the following elements:

1. *Biological or structural invariants.* In the case of an individual, this would be age, sex, and relevant structural information such as temperament, height, weight, and biological or medical strengths and liabilities. In the case of a school system, the physical nature of the buildings and their surroundings would be important.

2. *Developmental history.* I prefer a brief review of the primary events of the first few stages, using Erikson's framework.

3. *Current circumstances of the individual or family.*

4. *Coping maneuvers.* How is the individual or family responding to the interaction of elements 1 through 3.

There are two types of coping maneuvers: adaptive and maladaptive. Maladaptive maneuvers can be subdivided into those that are still reversible and those that have become irreversible. For example, transient stress reactions and temporary balance bargains, no matter how expedient and expensive, are reversible if they are not yet rigid enough to merit being designated a disease. If a maladaptive coping maneuver has become irreversibly ingrained in the individual or family dynamics, a formal differential diagnosis may apply.

Note that a formal diagnosis is only this last small portion of an overall formulation. In my opinion, a formulation is particularly useful when working with child-family problems. Psychiatric diagnoses of children are not only difficult but often unfair, if not dangerous, since we cannot confidently predict the direction of an organism's development. The extent to which maladaptive coping mechanisms have been irreversibly incorporated into the developing personality structure is a crucial distinction.

Guidelines for Use of Clinical Data

Having been so outspoken in criticizing the diagnostic process, what constructive suggestions do I have to offer? Although psychiatric diagnosis presents unsolved problems (Panzetta, 1974), I suggest the following guidelines for use of clinical data.

1. Collect the data as objectively as possible while maintaining maximum empathy with the patient.

2. After collecting a good data base, take a break before plunging into a diagnosis/formulation and try to clear your head of preconceptions.

3. Examine your data. Be prepared to throw out most of it. (It is amazing how agonizing this process can be!) Differentiate between news (something you did not know before) and data (information that generates some leverage on the problem facing you). Then consider the independent pieces of information that seem to bear on the clinical problem. The key word here is *independent* because we can place the greatest emphasis on patterns that are consistently reported and observed in different circumstances. (Campbell & Stanley, 1963).

4. Use whatever data is available to rule out critical possibilities. The following examples illustrate the crucial distinction between data that support an hypothesis and data that exclude a hypothesis. A distraught mother requested an evaluation of her seven-year-old son after another physician had looked at the child briefly and stated "He's autistic." When the child entered my office, he glanced around the room, looked me in the eye, and asked: "Can I play with your toys?" The first clinician may have observed a host of unusual behaviors—any one of which may have been consistent with a diagnosis of autism. However, one critical piece of information I was privileged to obtain rigorously excluded the diagnosis of autism, regardless of other behaviors I may have observed. Similarly, if you whisper softly to a child whose back is turned to you, "Eddy, do you suppose I have some candy in this drawer?" and the child immediately turns around and runs to your desk to search for the candy, you have ruled out the possibility of deafness. You have *not*, however, ruled out the possi-

bility of a temporary disruption in his state of consciousness, which might occur in petit mal epilepsy.

5. Construct a formulation that summarizes essential biological, developmental, and circumstantial facts and creates a context for a discussion of the individual's adaptive and maladaptive behaviors. Maladaptive behaviors can be subdivided into reversible and irreversible behaviors, and it is the *irreversible* maladaptive behaviors that provide the basis for a differential diagnosis.

6. If diagnosis is necessary, make a differential diagnosis: i.e., rank the reasonable diagnostic possibilities—including the data on which the diagnostic impressions rest and preferably some estimate of your confidence in the diagnostic impressions—in the order of their probability. I prefer to use the diagnostic categories proposed in *Psychopathological Disorders in Childhood* (Group for the Advancement of Psychiatry, 1966).

7. When dealing with difficult and confusing cases, the following rules are helpful: First, be extremely cautious, keeping in mind that the reliability of data and the validity of a diagnosis are probably low. Second, focus on the functional aspects of the problem: e.g., will the school counselor need a letter from you to obtain special tutoring for the child? To maximize the administrative and therapeutic effects of the appropriate diagnostic label while minimizing possible hazards, it may be worthwhile to discuss the label with a source of referral such as the school, which has a specific administrative use for such a label; with the parents; and preferably with the children. Third, it is wise, especially when a child has already been blessed with a number of formal diagnoses, to list

the diagnoses for which the child is *at risk* and, if possible, any strong evidence that excludes these diagnoses. Certain children seem to fall into a large category that can be called "at risk for being labeled hyperactive, brain damaged, emotionally disturbed, learning disorder, mentally retarded, maybe schizophrenic, possibly autistic, other." In these cases especially, one of our main responsibilities is to protect the child from the inevitable onslaught of the labeling process. When working with these youngsters, I prefer to rely heavily on the category called developmental deviation (Group for the Advancement of Psychiatry, 1966). One can then discuss the specific dimensions of development in which a deviation is observed and avoid global labels such as schizophrenic. The 1966 version of the GAP manual includes motor, sensory, speech, cognitive, social, psychosexual, affective, and integrative dimensions. This kind of description can be used with minimal trauma to parents and with minimal risk to the identified patient.

8. When dealing with a difficult diagnostic problem, it is appropriate to avoid a prediction, or the appearance of a prediction, and to make every effort to see the identified patient often enough to gain a long-term perspective about his development. When I discuss the concept of developmental deviation with distraught parents, I usually say: "He is on his own developmental course, and the usual kinds of predictions that we make about children may not apply." This statement can be followed by a discussion about the best course of action.

9. If one is in a position to observe the child's developmental course or response to therapy, it is preferable to review the data base and formulation and

then modify the formulation and diagnostic impression accordingly.[3]

In my opinion, the problem of diagnosis in psychiatry in general and in child psychiatry in particular is in a state of flux. Therefore, I have proposed a series of ground rules for handling data that are relevant to child-family problems. A formulation that involves important biological, developmental, and environmental factors may help to illuminate discussions about both adaptive and maladaptive behaviors currently observed. Relatively irreversible maladaptive behaviors may merit a differential diagnosis.

A final point about the use of data. Earlier, I mentioned that there is always the danger that we will become lazy and not do the work required to make a series of genuinely independent observations and thus lose the noise-reducing power of a series of independent observations.

A second hazard, and possibly a greater one, looms in staff conferences because an analysis of the data may reflect the staff's pecking order rather than the nature of the case material. This is particularly true concerning complex, multiproblem cases, which involve difficulties on the biological, psychological, family, and social levels. If a multiproblem family presents a somewhat different picture to different staff members, the stage is set for a conflict among staff. For example, consider the following situation. The identified patient presents a number of neurological "soft signs," a reading disability that may or may not have a biological basis, and a customary coping strategy that would commonly be described as "personality disorder, passive-aggressive type." The family picture is complicated by alcoholism; the fact that the child is the last of many; and, on the social level, a poor relationship with the neighborhood and the school. When dealing with this type of family, mental health staff are prone to dissipate their energies by pulling and tugging on different pieces of the case. The important point here is that data which will rigorously rule out a large number of possibilities are lacking and there are abundant data which are compatible with a number of possibilities. Furthermore, it is impossible to determine which point in the system is primarily causal since biological, psychological, family, and social factors reverberate back and forth to generate a confusing picture. A clear formulation in these cases is of the utmost importance, and diagnoses become dangerous. The staff pecking order may well replace more differentiated and sophisticated problem-solving modalities as the method of choice. Therefore, a chart that specifies strengths, liabilities, target problems, and plans at the biological, psychological, family, and social levels encourages useful discussions about complicated cases.

Obviously, we must collect our data before designing a formulation and recommending a treatment plan. Our problem is that we have enormous amounts of news (new information) and limited amounts of hard data that bear directly on the core of the case. The clinical challenge is to make strong inferences from data that can be obtained with minimal expenditure of time and energy. At best, the data-collection process will strengthen rather than tax the working alliance.

The use of data is enormously complex. Studies of decision-making in the face of uncertainty indicate that the human mind is not especially adept at making good judgments based on complex data. The presence of irrelevant information causes our judgment to deteriorate. Therefore, we must handle clinical data with care, realizing our limitations and the implications of psychiatric labels.

The next five chapters are organized around the evaluative outline that ends this chapter. The exceptionally dedicated student may want to use the entire outline with a few cases. Although I strongly recommend this procedure, I realize that the busy practitioner will never carry it out.

Evaluative Outline for Work with Families

I. Introductory Information (Chapter 3)

A. Identifying Data
Name, sex, date of birth, major psychiatric history of each family member. Family's address, telephone number, socioeconomic group, national origin. Date of first visit; date of current writeup. Other significant information.

B. Source of Referral

C. Sources of Information

D. Examiner's View of Family's Request for Evaluation

E. Previous Therapists

II. Current Behavioral Picture (Chapter 3)

A. Chief Complaints of the Child, Parents, Others

B. History of the Problem
1. What precipitated the current crisis?
2. Have any shifts occurred recently in the child's or family's life?
3. How did the symptoms evolve?

C. Healthy Behavioral Patterns of the Child, Parents, Others

D. Child's Strengths and Level of Functioning
1. General adaptability
2. School behavior
3. Social behavior

E. Family Circumstances: Financial and Social

III. Backgound of the Problem (Chapter 4)

A. Family and Social System: The Family Tree

B. Parents' Developmental Histories

C. Development of the Marriage and Family

    D. Family's Medical History: Acute and Chronic Illnesses

IV. Child's Developmental History (Chapter 5)

    A. Pregnancy
        1. Mother's physical and emotional health
        2. Parental attitudes and expectations

    B. Delivery

    C. Infancy
        1. Health
        2. Temperamental type
        3. Early parent-child interactions
        4. Shifts in parental attitudes

    D. Developmental Landmarks
        1. Physical growth
        2. Psychological growth

    E. Evolution of Personality

    D. Interactional Factors: Evolution of Role and Self-image
        1. Interactions with family
        2. Other interactions
        3. History of life trauma

    E. Medical History

V. Clinical Observations (Chapter 6)

    A. Family's Behavior in the Waiting Room

    B. Child's Behavior in the Office or Playroom
        1. Separation from parents
        2. Appearance, behavior, and attitude
        3. Temperamental type
        4. Problem-solving style: cognitive and interpersonal
        5. Behavior during interviews
        6. Thought processes and language structure

   7. Affect
   8. Motor skills
   9. Memory
  10. Perception and perceptual-motor skills

  D. Family's Behavior During Conjoint Sessions
   1. Major roles and patterns
   2. Communication: major content and process
   3. Patterns of identification: alliances and barriers
   4. Four parameters of family function
   5. Affect
   6. Problem-solving style

  E. Parents' Behavior

  F. Others in the Social Network

  G. Additional Sources of Data

VI. Case Formulation and Treatment Plan (Chapter 7)
  A. Evaluating the Identified Patient
   1. Temperamental type
   2. GAP and DSM=II classifications
   3. Psychosexual development: optimal and predominant levels of functioning
   4. Major identifications and introjections
   5. Genetic-dynamic factors: major intrapsychic conflicts and their developmental origins
   6. Economic factors: distribution and availability of intrapsychic resources
   7. Major assets and liabilities: biological, psychological, family, and social-institutional

  B. Evaluating the Family
   1. The family as a system
    a. Rules of adaptation related to Type I processes

        b. Rules of adaptation related to Type II processes

        c. Roles and family mythology

        d. Communication: clarity; adequacy in current crisis

        e. Problem-solving style

    2. The family as an environment

        a. Capacity to ensure physical survival

        b. Capacity to validate reality testing and affect

        c. Existence of covert agendas

        d. Capacity for intimacy

        e. Capacity to facilitate differentiation

        f. Existence of major alliances and barriers

C. Analysis of Current Symptoms

    1. Symptoms related to biological disorders

    2. Symptoms as adaptive responses

    3. Symptoms as maladaptive responses

    4. Syntonicity or dystonicity of symptoms for the child, family, others

D. Treatment Plan

    1. Specific target problems and interventions

    2. Special precautions

    3. Case summaries

NOTES

1. Although the opinions expressed in this section are my own, I wish to express my gratitude to Dr. Baruch Fischoff of the Oregon Research Institute for his helpful suggestions.
2. *Question:* "What did Tarzan say when the elephants came by with sunglasses on?"
   Answer: "He didn't recognize them, so he didn't say anything."
   Moral: Perhaps the observation of *sunglasses* leads to a premature rejection of the possibility of elephants.
3. I am indebted to Dr. Charlotte Cook for suggestions concerning this section and especially for bringing to my attention Paul Meehl's essay titled "Why I Do Not Attend Case Conferences."

Chapter 3

INTRODUCTORY INFORMATION AND CURRENT BEHAVIORAL PICTURE

INTRODUCTORY INFORMATION

Indentifying data. In addition to conventional data such as the name, age, and sex of the identified patient, any information that will be critical when evaluating subsequent data should be included in this initial section of the outline. For example, if the identified patient has just been released from a psychiatric facility, is taking high doses of antipsychotic medication, or is the child of a chaotic family with specific risk factors such as a recent divorce, this fact should be stated at the outset, although logically it should appear later in the outline.

Sources of referral. When you enter the source or sources of referral in the outline, make certain that you include specific names, addresses, and telephone numbers.

Sources of information. The names and telephone numbers of all individuals who supply information about the identified patient or his family should be listed. This kind of information tends to slip away and is difficult to retrieve. In some instances, the bias of another agency or therapist that has worked with the family might be included. A possible covert agenda on the part of another agency should also be noted. We are all familiar with the way difficult cases are sometimes dumped on other agencies!

Examiner's view of family's request for evaluation. Frequently, an examiner suspects that the family has a hidden agenda for requesting an evaluation. For example, if there is an impending legal battle concerning custody of children, the examiner is well advised to ask specifically whether a legal issue is active because the evaluation may be used as ammunition in the courtroom. In cases where the evaluation is carried out against the patient's wishes at the insistence of a third party such as a parole officer, it cannot proceed until the third party has been consulted. The problem here is one created by the wide disparity of power among different people. This issue will be discussed further in Chapters 6 and 8.

Previous therapists. This section should include the names and addresses of any previous therapists and, optimally, their reports on the identified patient or family. A borderline picture can be clarified diagnostically only by a reasonable period of therapy, as illustrated by the following case:

> A young man was referred to the clinic by his parents, who announced that because of his offensive attitude toward them, they preferred not to be involved in therapy. However, they described a ranch where their son had lived as a boy. When we contacted the director of the ranch, a psychologist, he, recalled Bill very well. Although Bill had lived there for about seven years and had established strong attachments to several members of the staff, he had never made lasting gains in therapy. Every time a staff member had left, Bill had regressed to his previous level of functioning. They had tried "every medicine in the book" without success.

CURRENT BEHAVIORAL PICTURE

Chief Compaints

The simple point that a specific chief complaint is essential to a good workup cannot be overemphasized. If the complaint is unclear, the workup will proceed in a similar manner. It may be useful to reestablish the chief complaint periodically; I usually do this at the end of the workup because it is not uncommon for the initial complaint to shift markedly during the several sessions involved in the evaluation.

When evaluating young children, I prefer to see the identified patient and his parents together during the initial session and ask them fairly broad questions such as "What kinds of problems do you want us to help you with?" Commonly, the parents indicate that they feel uncomfortable about discussing important issues in the child's presence. In response, I usually tell them to "Talk about things to the extent that you're comfortable." My objective in saying this is not only to gain specific information about the family's chief complaints but to see how the child-parent system handles the problems that are inherent in the interview.

When the identified patient is an adolescent, however, I always see him alone first and then ask his parents to join us. It is essential, when working with adolescents, to clarify the primary working relationship. If the primary alliance is to be between the therapist and the parents, this must be made clear to everyone at the outset. If the primary alliance is to be with the adolescent, this fact must be discussed explicitly with the parents. To share with parents information that has been obtained in confidence from the adolescent is, of course, disastrous, and the adolescent will anticipate (often correctly) that the therapist has been brought in as a powerful ally of the parents to resolve a family struggle. These issues must be clarified at the beginning.

Chief complaints are best reported as direct quotations. Note in the outline that the chief complaints include those of the identified patient, the parents, and other key figures because disparities often reveal crucial information about the nature of the problem. For example, the father may insist that "The child always lies to us and we can never make him mind," while the identified patient's chief complaint may be: "My father always beats me, no matter what I do." The school may report, on the other hand, that "The parents have no end of excuses to keep him out of school." It is critical to the success of the subsequent evaluation and therapy to consider each individual's chief complaint, not only on its own merits but as part of the overall picture. Because it is tempting to take the side of the family member whose suffering most clearly matches the examiner's, it is essential for the sake of the working alliance to recognize and acknowledge the validity of each individual chief complaint and explore the disparities between them.

In later chapters I will elaborate extensively on the point that a family which comes for an evaluation is almost always involved in a power struggle (see especially, Chapter 8). As a result, family members may anxiously watch the new element in the system—the therapist—to see whether he will function as an ally of one person or another. Therefore, the therapist must handle direct questions about the "rightness" or "wrongness" of certain behaviors with care, especially at the outset, until he has developed a working alliance with both the identified patient and the entire family system.

History of the Problem

The process by which symptoms have evolved is one of our best sources of information about the family structure. We are especially interested in any evidence bearing on the syntonic-dystonic distinction. For example, is the problem acute? Are there clear precipitating factors? Have the symptoms fluctuated? Do family members take turns being ill? Satir (1971) emphasized the value of finding out who first labeled the symptoms and how the perception that a family member was symptomatic then became part of the family process. Bowen (1966) pointed out that two individuals who are experiencing severe stress will try to reduce that stress by involving a third person. According to Bowen, a family has three options for managing stress: marital dysfunction, illness or dysfunction on the part of a parent, or illness or dysfunction in one of the children. The development of symptoms within the family system therefore indicates the kind of homeostatic maneuver that the family will use as it responds to excessive stress. Do family members characteristically develop psychosomatic symptoms in times of stress? Do they plunge into bouts of alcoholism or abusive behavior? Do the family roles characteristically become increasingly rigid and does the family attempt to use only Type I maneuvers during stress? Or can it make adaptive shifts in its reference system? Boszormenyi-Nagy and Spark (1973) delineated the important fact that coping patterns are transmitted from one generation to the next (see also, Mendell & Fisher, 1956; Tomas, 1969).

As I mentioned in Chapter 1, we are extremely interested in the degree of reversibility of the symptoms. For example, we are often concerned about the distinction between an adjustment reaction in a healthy child and family, which by definition is reversible and transient, and a developmental deviation (See Group for the Advancement of Psychiatry, 1966), in which loss of reversibility is a serious consideration and therefore may indicate the need for therapy. When making this distinction, knowing how the symptoms developed is extremely useful. Obviously, if specific symptoms appear abruptly following an identifiable stress, the prognosis is more encouraging because the symptoms suggest an adjustment reaction. In contrast, maladaptive patterns between parents and child which develop gradually over a period of years and are arbitrarily labeled as symptoms at some point should make us suspect that the symptoms are deeply embedded in the family dynamics. Generally speaking, if the family gives evidence of role-rigidity in the form of a fixed sequence of communication (Haley, 1967) or wide discrepancies between feeling tone, verbal and behavioral communications, and so on, it is fairly safe to assume that the family system is protecting itself from the enormous amount of energy the family believes would be required to make a Type II shift. (Chapter 8 describes how the clinician can obtain a rough estimate of the turbulence involved in the rearrangement required for a Type II shift.) Frequently, the fact that a family presents itself for evaluation reflects the family's threshold of tolerance for a particular type of behavior, not the severity or increase in severity of symptoms observed by an outsider.

WHAT PRECIPITATED THE CURRENT CRISIS?   By determining the specific factors that precipitated the family's request for help, we can learn much about the family's rules of adaptation. Families enter the mental health system by numerous routes. If pressure from an outside agency is the precipitating event, as is often the case, the family will behave differently from one that actively seeks help. The precipitating event is often an eloquent illustration of how the family defines acceptable and unacceptable behavior.

> Mr. and Mrs. N brought their 14-year-old son, Bob, to the Crisis Clinic and demanded hospitalization or long-term residential placement. Mr. N reported that his son was violent and dangerous and refused to take Bob home. It soon became clear that pitched battles between father and son had been going on for years and that the current crisis was precipitated by Bob's spurt of growth at puberty. As Bob put it: "For years, we had these fights and I was always on the

floor. Now, for once, *he's* flat on the floor, so I'm all of a sudden crazy!"

Obviously, this type of aggressive behavior would concern any parent, but the context in which the behavior occurs might lead us to question whether there is a family rule that it is acceptable for Mr. N to hit his son, verbally or otherwise, but the reverse is unacceptable. Furthermore, is there a larger rule that Mr. N has the right to rule. In other words, is Bob challenging the first and obvious set of rules (You're not allowed to hit your dad) as well as a larger set (Only dad gets to write really important rules). Based on the presenting picture, it would be impossible to determine whether the family's anxiety is related to Bob's physical aggression or to the possibility that the family is faced with a significant restructuring as a result of Bob's entry into adolescence. The clinical objective, of course, is to raise questions—as gracefully and appropriately as possible—about the family's power structure while acknowledging the painful feelings involved. For example:

> Sixteen-year-old Ed was brought to the Crisis Clinic in a withdrawn catatonic state. The family's chief complaint was that he had said, "I heard a voice." A history revealed that Ed had been standing quietly near a wall most of the time for two or three years whenever he was at home. His parents attributed this to his overhearing a statement that he was an adopted child. His response to this statement had been: "Well, if you're not my family, I'm not going to talk to you people again." Although the family had not considered Ed's standing motionless next to a wall for hours as particularly unusual, it was most disturbed by his hallucination.

The two examples just cited involved families who were propelled into the mental health system by a sizable crisis. Other families, however, may perceive themselves as severely stressed over a period of years and find their way into therapy in a somewhat more fortuitous manner. For instance, parents who have had the opportunity to discuss a problem informally with a mental health worker after a PTA meeting may feel comfortable enough to seek therapy, but only on the condition that they can see that particular therapist. There is no specific precipitating event; yet the mode of entry clearly signals the family's anxiety about the possibility of trauma at the hands of a therapist.

This type of situation should warn the clinician that the family feels extremely vulnerable to the stress that might occur as the family mythology is examined!

HAVE ANY RECENT SHIFTS OCCURRED IN THE CHILD'S OR FAMILY'S LIFE?   Most clinicans are unaware of, or are slow to acknowledge the traumatic impact of what an outsider may view as ordinary events. Patients are carefully trained to present to the professional healer only those wounds that are obvious and severe enough to merit respect and concern. However, the accumulation of numerous small wounds within a certain period may lead to a breakdown of the system. The task of evaluation is complicated by at least two factors: (1) the stress value of life events is highly idiosyncratic and (2) individuals vary widely in terms of how much stress they can handle within a certain period. The task of evaluating children is even more complicated because adults are reluctant to accept the fact that a child can and does suffer intensely because of the magical nature of his logical structure and because of his limited ability to communicate his perception of the world in verbal terms. Coddington (1972a and b) pointed out that a wide variety of events have a significant stress value for children and that the accumulation of stresses within a given period will generate symptoms.

HOW DID THE SYMPTOMS EVOLVE?   Framo (1970) delineated a variety of events that commonly generate symptoms within the family structure: e.g., irrational assignment of roles, blurring of generational boundaries, and changes in the family relationship system. To his credit, Framo also pointed out that "just as there are symptoms which insure one thing in the family system, preventing true individuation, so there are symptoms which are designed to help get one out of the system [p. 282]." We can summarize Framo's important points in the Type I- Type II terms outlined in Chapter 1. Framo discussed Type II issues and processes in every case; that is, he emphasized that disease results when there is a problem with the reference system or mythology with respect to which the family is functioning. "Conscious, formal, instrumental family roles, described by sociologists, are not under discussion here because they are not very pertinent to psychopathology; it is the discrepancy between the irrational, informal role assignment and the natural family role that creates the difficulties [p. 274]." Clearly, this is a Type II issue, as we have defined it, since the identified patient is trying to relate simultaneously to two separate reference systems. Type II confusion guarantees chaos. This is not surprising if we remember that the mythology, which establishes the roles, serves the same essential function for the family organism that physiological reference points serve at the biological level. If a system lacks reference points, chaos is inevitable because neither Type I nor Type II processes can take place.

The following cases illustrate the three major types of events that can generate symptoms in the family:

Irrational assignment of roles. Six-year-old Billie had been rejected by his family since birth. Both his sisters were wanted children. His parents said they had not wanted a third child, but "if we had to have a third child, we wanted it to be a girl." With respect to Billie's sex, his mother casually remarked: "Well, if he wanted to have that sex change operation someday, that would be O.K. with me—of course, it would be entirely up to him." When, after two years of therapy, the

family accepted Billie as a male, one of his sisters became
severely symptomatic.

Blurring of generational boundaries. Preadolescent Jim was unable to function in school despite his good intelligence. The
family consisted of Jim and his mother; he had never known
his father. His general pattern was one of extremely passive-
aggressive behavior such as not turning in his school assign-
ments on time. At home, his interactions with his mother
reflected considerable confusion about whether he should
relate to her as a small child, an adolescent male, or an adult.
At least part of Jim's floundering in school was related to his
attempts to obtain a clear definition of generational boun-
dries.

Changes in the family relationship system. Mr. and Mrs. Z developed severe marital difficulties in late middle age after their
eldest daughter left home at an appropriate age. In response
to these difficulties, Mrs. Z left her husband. He immediately
developed a series of serious illnesses, and she returned
home to care for him. Presumably the Zs correctly perceived
that the shifts which were occurring were not simply routine
oscillations within the family's role system (a Type I process)
but were significant challenges to the family roles and belief
structure: i.e., their daughter's departure forced a series of
Type II changes within the family, which resulted in marital
problems and illness.

Usually, the family views the identified patient's symptoms as arising spontaneously from within him, totally
apart from general family processes. For example, parents
often say with considerable emotion: "He just does those
things for no reason whatever!" (See the section in this
chapter dealing with the coherence of the chief complaint.)
Usually, however, we can assume that any persistent pattern of behavior is related in some way to the family's basic
structure. This is by no means the same as saying that the
family makes the child sick or keeps the child sick. The
family, like any organism, must respond to strong forces

within it, and the direction of causality—from child to family and from family to child—must be carefully evaluated in each case. In this process, the family history is one of our most useful tools.

In summary, understanding how the symptoms evolved helps us to understand whether they are syntonic or dystonic. Cases that merit professional attention almost invariably involve symptoms that have developed over a relatively long period and have some significance in the general process of family adaptation. Therefore, it is crucially important to obtain as much information as possible about how the symptoms evolved. The following case illustrates this point:

> Mrs. A insisted that her 12-year-old son, Sam, was hyperactive, and she refused all forms of evaluation except those required to prescribe medication. She and Mr. A were divorced and never interacted except when she called him about Sam's misbehavior. Gradually it became clear that the boy's misbehavior provided the parents with a reason to communicate with each other. Although they were unwilling to acknowledge it to themselves or to each other, their son's symptoms were mutually beneficial to them and protected them from having to acknowledge the depth of their interest in one another. In other words, they were trying to violate the law that there is no free lunch.

Healthy Behavioral Patterns

Behavioral clinicians focus on pathology to the exclusion of healthy behavior to a degree that sometimes borders on the pathologically coprophilic. Must we remain blind to the fact that our patients (individuals or families) do have conflict-free areas of functioning? We have no difficulty believing that family members are capable of making each other ill. Is it impossible to believe that they can make each other well? During our somber reflections about pathology, can't we acknowledge the reality of love and joy? As I review this manuscript, I find that I have focused almost exclusively on the grim aspects of family life. Such is the selective bias of the clinician. Generally speaking, a diagnosis refers only to one area of a persons's life; yet because psychiatric diagnoses have a far greater splatter effect than biological ones, they tend to create a global and negative value judgment. The purpose of the following examples is to illustrate how different family members normally spend their time.

> *Identified patient.* Dick functions extremely well in his adolescent peer group, maintains long-term friendships, and is a loyal and considerate friend. The symptomatic behaviors for which his parents request residential treatment (smoking marijuana, drinking, and sexual activity) are normal in the context of his peer group.

> *Parents.* Dick's parents have enjoyed their marriage. They share an active interest in a number of spectator sports and attend sports events throughout the year.

Child's Strengths and Level of Functioning

An overall assessment of the child's adaptability, social behavior, and school performance often tells us about his ability to cope with stress and the kinds of symptoms that are likely to emerge when stress becomes excessive.

GENERAL ADAPTABILITY.   We may be able to obtain some historical information about the identified patient's general ability to handle crises and to take active advantage of opportunities. Obviously, this information bears heavily on the differential diagnosis, prognosis, and treatment plans. For example:

> Six-year-old Ann came to the attention of the school psychologist because she seemed withdrawn, apathetic, and distant, interacted minimally with her peers, and produced almost no school work. If another child hit her on the play-

ground, she seemed confused rather than aggressive or angry. In fact, she rarely showed evidence of emotion. Her
parents confirmed that Ann's behavior at school was consistent with her behavior at home; she also behaved this way
in the clinical setting.

In Ann's case, the differential diagnosis was extremely
broad, and the evaluation had to include a consideration of
biological, psychological, family, and social factors.

> Mr. and Mrs. B described their eight-year-old son's behavior
> as extremely hyperactive and obnoxious. However, Mrs. B
> noted with some irritation that "When he's at the neigh-
> bor's, he is just an ideal boy, and he seems really happy."
> The clinician observed that the boy was often cheerful and
> symptom free but immediately became angry whenever he
> became involved in any kind of power struggle.

SCHOOL BEHAVIOR.   The massive series of experiences
subsumed under the heading "school" tests a child's perceptual, motor, affective, cognitive, interpersonal, and integrative abilities. Therefore, a youngster who functions well
in all areas of school is unlikely to exhibit serious pathology. Conversely, a youngster who does poorly in school
may be normal, bright, or suffering from any kind of disorder. Thus the specificity of information gained from poor
school functioning is low. The sensitivity of school person-
nel is variable. Although the staff usually reacts strongly to
the disruptive child, the quietly depressed or psychiatrically
borderline student may slide through year after gradually
decompensating year. In any case, the therapist should at
least telephone the school—after obtaining the permission
of the child and his parents.

Because the assessment of academic function has been
discussed in detail by other authors (e.g., Ilg & Ames, 1964;
Long & Morse, 1965; Scagliotto, 1970; Thorndike & Hagen, 1955), the focus here is on interpersonal problems, of
which school difficulties may be only a symptom. For exam-

ple, does the child always respond well to teachers of one sex and poorly to teachers of the other sex? The distinction between *can't* and *won't* is not only crucial operationally but is a useful focus for organizing both the workup and discussions with parents.[1]

> Eleven-year-old Larry was doing well in school, except in math, which had been easy for him in previous years. It soon became apparent that his problems were related to a power struggle with his teacher, which was displaced from intrafamilial conflict. Therefore, Larry's uneven functioning led the clinician to look carefully at the specific interactions between Larry and the math teacher and at Larry's tendency to overreact to her.

SOCIAL BEHAVIOR.   Although the child's capacity to play and therefore to relate in a healthy way to his peers is essential for normal cognitive development (Piers, 1975), the psychoanalytic model emphasizes the importance of the child's progressive ability to invest his libido outside the immediate nuclear family. H. R. Huessy observed a significant difference between children who have maintained at least one friendship for six months or more and children who have been unable to do so (personal communication, Miami, Florida, May 1976). Generally speaking, the difference between a complete lack of friends and one lasting friendship is far greater than the difference between one friendship and many.[2] Examination of the child's peer relationships is, of course, crucial if the differential diagnosis includes schizophrenia or a personality disorder of the schizoid type. The presence of one enduring friendship demonstrates unequivocally that the child is capable of establishing a mutually satisfying, ongoing relationship with another person.

The child's relationships with teachers and administrators indicates his ability to relate to authority figures. In this context, Erikson's Eight Ages of Man are useful when attempting to determine whether a child's school difficulties reflect intrapsychic conflict. Do his recurrent problems seem to involve issues related to Stage 1, for example? Does the child participate in activities such as Scouting or Little League? His capacity to function within a permanent, structured situation demonstrates his degree of adaptability, social competence, and so forth.

Family Circumstances

Although the child lives and develops in the context of a family, family members may underestimate the significance of their circumstances and leave the clinician to ferret out the relevant information. Similarly, family members may underestimate the importance of illnesses and other major drains on the family's energy. Subtle shifts in the relationships among family members may escape notice or be hidden deliberately.

> The B family lives in a lower middle-class neighborhood that is crowded with children, dogs, motorcycles, and nonfunctional pickup trucks. Their neighbor has vowed to react immediately and violently if any member of the B family sets foot on his property. Fights between the two families' dogs are frequent and lead to serious threats. In this setting, the identified patient's misbehavior is dangerous.

> Fourteen-year-old Mary was reticent to talk. Her upper middle-class parents had dropped her off at the clinic, hoping to hear later from the clinician what was wrong with her. Mary had become sullen, withdrawn, and uncooperative during the school year. The fact that approximately 12 months before, her mother had returned to work after years of child-rearing represented a major crisis for this family. The mother's new-found personal and financial autonomy tipped the balance of a carefully and deeply concealed marital conflict and triggered her husband into drinking bouts and sexual promiscuity. This key information emerged late in the fourth session, prefaced with "Of course this has nothing to do with it, but. . . ."

NOTES

1. My thanks to Pat Staling, teacher of special education, for her helpful comments.
2. This distinction between zero and one is useful in many areas of evaluation. In general, one event unequivocally demonstrates the system's capacity, as a boundary condition, to hold a particular configuration. As a result, the basis for the *rarity* of that configuration can be explored in detail. This is different from *zero*, for in this case we do not know whether the system has within its boundary conditions the capacity to attain a particular configuration. Clinically, it appears that a 0–1 distinction is enormously important, a 1–2 distinction is usually important, and a 2–10 distinction is probably but not necessarily important. These details may be relevant to a wide variety of clinical phenomena: e.g., "He never pays any attention to me," "The children always act badly at grandma's." "Nothing I *ever* do turns out well."

Chapter 4

BACKGROUND OF THE PROBLEM

Although collecting data about an individual's physical structure and functioning is one of the oldest traditions in the medical profession, the practice of collecting data that are useful in assessing family structure and functioning is still in its infancy. One exciting area in family theory is the multigenerational transmission of behavior patterns. In a pioneering paper titled "An Approach to Neurotic Behavior in Terms of a Three Generation Family Model," Mendell and Fisher discussed the development of a patient's symptoms in terms of their restorative value for the family. In 1966 Bowen emphasized "the survey of the family fields" as the basis for evaluating family function, and Minuchin (1974) developed a detailed method of analyzing family structure and function. Boszormenyi-Nagy and Spark have discussed the importance of family structure extensively in their book *Invisible Loyalties.*

FAMILY AND SOCIAL SYSTEM: THE FAMILY TREE

The family tree is an extremely useful tool for obtaining a concise summary of a wealth of critical information about the structure of the family and social system. In addition, essential information about how the family and social system function can be indicated by noting which members hold the most power and how they view the family situation (Satir, 1971; Bowen, 1966). These two types of information —family composition and the predominant mythology or belief structure—go a long way toward giving the clinician a detailed psychological map of the family. This information not only describes the terrain where the identified patient dwells and functions, it allows us to draw inferences about important clinical events in his developmental history, such as the birth of siblings.

Degree of differentiation can be compared in this analogy to the *steepness* of the terrain. To deviate even slightly from the predominant mythology (lateral movement), a *poorly* differentiated family must do a large amount of work (vertical movement) because Type II processes consume an enormous amount of energy. A better differentiated family is able to shift roles more easily. The analogy to a three-dimensional, topographic map is therefore relatively direct. The poorly differentiated family behaves as though it lives in a deep valley: to move out of the valley is difficult and possibly hazardous. Consequently, family members tend to stay close to home (physically or in terms of belief structure). If they do break away, they tend to erect a strong barrier between themselves and the family of origin and often become enmeshed in the mythology of a "rescuing" family!

In summary, the family tree outlines the basic family *structure*, the predominant *mythology*, and the family's level of *differentiation*. By combining this information, it is possible to create a topographical map of the identified patient's environment.

The ordinal position of children within the family has been studied extensively and is a rich source of valuable, easily collected data (Toman, 1969). If no more than sibling position and sex of the identified patient is available, useful generalizations can be made about family patterns, especially if the family is not well differentiated. For this reason, it is often useful to include information about as many generations as possible.

Figure 4.1 contains a list of symbols that make it possible to summarize the family structure in a single chart. Figure 4.2 illustrates how these symbols can be combined to indicate current and former marriages or alliances and their duration, separations and divorces, ages of siblings, composition of the parents' families of origin, the current living and social units, and so forth. (Note that temperamental type, cause of death, and other facts are easily incorporated into this system.) In addition, the major mythology, particularly as it concerns the identified patient and his symptoms, can be briefly described, ideally in the form of quotations, with speaker and referent clearly indicated.

Figure 4.3 illustrates a typical family, the Rollas. Lowell, the identified patient, is four years, two months old. He lives with his mother, age 23, stepfather, age 28; and half-brother, Freddie, age two years and two months. He has never met his biological father. Lowell has had a difficult temperament since birth. Freddie, on the other hand, has always exhibited an easy temperament.

The extended family includes Mrs. Rolla's parents and three sisters. Mrs. Rolla is the fourth of five children. Her father, age 50, is a reformed alcoholic. Her mother, also 50 years old, wields the power in the family; she not only establishes the roles of family members but insists that the members adhere to them. (Information about the three

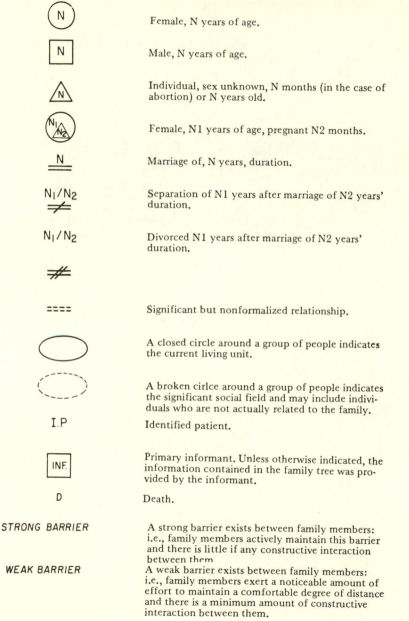

Female, N years of age.

Male, N years of age.

Individual, sex unknown, N months (in the case of abortion) or N years old.

Female, N1 years of age, pregnant N2 months.

Marriage of, N years, duration.

Separation of N1 years after marriage of N2 years' duration.

Divorced N1 years after marriage of N2 years' duration.

Significant but nonformalized relationship.

A closed circle around a group of people indicates the current living unit.

A broken cirlce around a group of people indicates the significant social field and may include individuals who are not actually related to the family.

Identified patient.

Primary informant. Unless otherwise indicated, the information contained in the family tree was provided by the informant.

Death.

A strong barrier exists between family members: i.e., family members actively maintain this barrier and there is little if any constructive interaction between them

A weak barrier exists between family members: i.e., family members exert a noticeable amount of effort to maintain a comfortable degree of distance and there is a minimum amount of constructive interaction between them.

Figure 4.1   Basic Symbols for Constructing the Family Tree

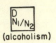
(alcoholism)

This person died of alcoholism N1 years ago at the age of N2.

Easy, Slow-to-warm
Difficult

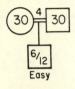
Easy

A couple, both partners 30 years old, have been married four years and have a six-month-old son with an easy temperament.

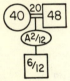

A couple married 20 years; he is 48, she is 40. Their son, adopted at age two months, is now six months old.

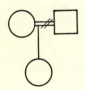

Parents are divorced; mother has custody of daughter.

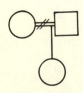

Parents are divorced; father has custody of daughter.

Figure 4.2   Family Trees Constructed of the Basic Symbols

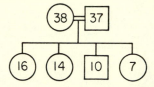

Ordinal position of siblings is indicated by arranging children according to age.

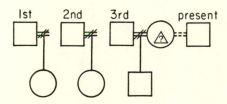

A woman has been married three times and now lives with a man by whom she is pregnant. She has custody of a daughter by each of the first two marriages and a son by the third.

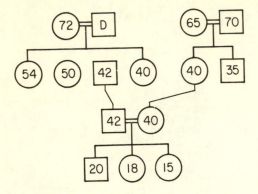

To reduce crowding and confusion, the identified patient's parents can be entered twice. This diagram uses four horizontal rows to chart three generations: rows two and three both indicate the identified patient's parents.

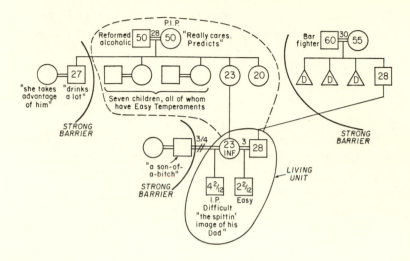

Figure 4.3   The Rolla Family Tree

aunts, if relevant, could be included in the chart and in the narrative.)

Mr. Rolla is an only child, born after three unsuccessful pregnancies. He refuses to communicate with his family of origin.

The chart also includes significant statements about Lowell and other family members and comments about the level of differentiation. In addition, it indicates problems of special interest. First, the maternal grandfather's history of alcoholism raises the possibility that Mrs. Rolla has learned a pattern of intimacy based on illness-rescue maneuvers (see Berne, 1964). If this is the case, Lowell will be prone to strong pressures to be dysfunctional so that the family will have someone to rescue. Second, as the unwanted reminder of an unhappy marriage who is now displaced by the True Son, Lowell is in an extremely vulnerable position. This problem is severely exacerbated by his difficult temperament, which contrasts sharply with Freddie's easygoing temperament. Third, Freddie was born when

Lowell was two—an age when the conflict between the wish for intimacy and the wish for autonomy is especially active. The appearance of the threatening half-sibling at this point could complicate the resolution of this developmental problem. Fourth, the maternal grandmother's position as the person in power is extremely strong. She keeps close tabs on other family members. Furthermore, the others view her as the one who "really cares," which may complicate the task of thwarting her predictions. Mr. Rolla not only left his family of origin but erected a strong barrier between them. Yet, like any organism, he must have a reference structure and therefore is likely to be loyal to the belief structure of his wife's family. Because new converts to any faith are generally its most vociferous defenders, Mr. Rolla is likely to be a staunch ally of his mother-in-law as a fount of goodness and wisdom. For these reasons, the grandmother's adaptiveness, life history, and attitude toward Lowell are of great importance. Fifth, from the parents' ordinal possitions, we can obtain further information. Mr. Rolla is an only child, born when his mother was in her late twenties, after a series of miscarriages. His specialness as an only child is therefore intensified. However, the fact that he has left his own family and erected a strong barrier against it would lead us to surmise that some family patterns will appear intact in the next generation while other patterns that are assiduously avoided will appear in a "mirror image" form. Toman (1969) predicted that an only son "does not have much use for children except maybe for one that turns out to be the spitting image of himself [p. 116]." Therefore, it would be difficult for Mr. Rolla to develop a strong tie to a stepson, even in the best of circumstances.

The effects of Mrs. Rolla's position as the second of three daughters is less clear. However, we do know that she lacked good role models for males (e.g., if a strong, functional brother had been part of the family network, an alternative to the rescue relationship might have been possible). Therefore, a search of the family tree—and Mrs. Rolla's belief system—concerning the essential nature of males would be extremely worthwhile.

On the basis of all this information, we would expect the chief complaint to fall from the family tree like an over-ripe peach, and in fact, the family's major complaint was "Lowell hates his younger brother."

Figure 4.4 illustrates a poorly differentiated, multi-problem, chaotic family called the Smiths. A staff conference about a case like this is usually prefaced by "You won't BAH-LEEVE this family!" followed by a lengthy narrative that boggles the middle-class clinician's mind. But in essence these cases are basically simple: The label "chaotic, multiproblem, and poorly differentiated family of social class five" puts major constraints on the family system, which is highly predictable and stable in its chaos. Usually, all that is needed are a few specific sentences about the type of chaos (e.g., addiction or penal or psychiatric institutionalization). It is seldom worth the time and effort to construct a detailed family tree. Far more difficult is an analysis of the subtle interplay of forces in upper-class families that fight with verbal nuance rather than weapons. Thus a detailed family tree can be useful when working with these families.

A narrative description of the Smith family might sound something like this: The identified patient, Bobby Smith, age seven, lives with his 26-year-old mother; her fourth husband; two half-sisters, ages four and three, who are his mother's children by her second husband; and a two-year-old half-sister, his mother's child by her fourth husband. For all practical purposes, the current living unit also includes Mr. Smith's girlfriend and their four-year-old daughter, who live in the same tenement.

Mrs. Smith left home and married at age 16; after one year the marriage ended in divorce. The children of this marriage, two boys, ages 10 and 11, live elsewhere. At 18,

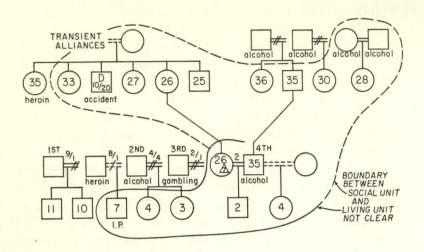

Figure 4.4 The Smith Family Tree

Mrs. Smith lived with but did not marry Bobby's father; she left him after a year when she discovered he was addicted to heroin. At age 19, she married her second husband, who was an alcoholic and the father of her four- and three-year-old daughters. Four years later she divorced him and married a hard-working tradesman who was a compulsive gambler. She divorced him a year later and married Mr. Smith, a 35-year-old alcoholic who is the father of Mrs. Smith's two-year-old son and his girlfriend's four-year-old daughter, who lives with the Smiths most of the time. The Smiths are expecting their second child in two months.

Mr. and Mrs. Smith have frequent and significant contacts with members of both extended families. Mrs. Smith's mother lives nearby and Bobby has always been her favorite grandchild. She never married; her five children were the result of transient alliances. Her 35-year-old daughter is a heroin addict and lives in another city. Her second daughter, age 33, lives nearby. Her son, who would now be 30, died ten years ago from injuries sustained in a car accident. Her third daughter, age 27, lives nearby. Her second son, age 25, is currently in prison for an assault that allegedly took place during an attempted armed robbery. His mother visits him whenever she can.

Mr. Smith is the second of four children and his mother's only son. His mother, father, and two stepfathers are alcoholics.

Bobby was referred by the school because of his frequent truancies and extremely poor academic performance. The teacher suspected he lacked motivation, while Mrs. Smith insisted that the school was overcrowded, unsafe, and staffed with poor teachers who "just don't know how to get kids interested."

PARENTS' DEVELOPMENTAL HISTORIES

The family tree can be extremely useful for evaluating the degree of congruency between behavioral patterns observed in the identified patient and those *reported* by the parents' about their own developmental histories. A word of caution is necessary here, however. Data obtained from parents are highly biased, having been subjected to selective recall, secondary elaboration, and so forth. Therefore, we do not obtain a history in a true sense; we obtain part of the *current version* of the individual's memories of previous life events, which may have only the most superficial relationship to his actual history.

Of what value, then, are these data? The answer is that they may be far more useful for our purposes than an "objective" history because they approximate the version of the individual's life history which is real to him—and that, after all, is the version that will have some bearing on his current behavior. Thus, although we must be aware of the enormous biases inherent in the situation, the problem is self-correcting to an extent.

A useful concept for integrating the parents' developmental histories with the identified patient's symptoms is that of intimacy or loyalty. The infant *has no option* but to pledge allegiance to the nuclear family's reference structure. And if this pledge involves the fulfillment of certain requirements, as it must, the child will be compelled to meet at least some parental expectations. Development can be viewed as a series of solutions to "mini-max" problems: i.e., the growing child seeks to *maximize* his loyalty to his family and his own intrinsic biological strivings while *minimizing* the amount of energy he must expend to do so. Individuals who are capable of mature intimacy find joy in the enormous variation in the human personality. Those who are less capable are threatened by it and seem unable to share their innermost experiences on a verbal level. Therefore, they are compelled to seek out another individual whose life appears to match their own, hoping to share an inner experience through the congruency of life patterns. If the environment does not provide an individual with the appropriate requirements, a second option is to "manufacture" one within the family. In other words, the basically healthy desire to share a deep and powerful life experience may cause a parent to reinforce certain behaviors in the child and thus create a life picture that is similar to his own. (See the discussion on balance bargains in Chapter 1.) This process may confront the parent with a cruel dilemma: should he suffer a deep sense of isolation concerning important experiences and therefore never experience full intimacy with another person? Or should he subject his child to the very agonies that he suffered in his own life? Although this process is relatively uniform from one family to another, the content varies as widely as that of other behavior. Thus the son who has had a long, brilliant professional career may be just as bound to the mythology of his family as is the unfortunate soul whose script requires addiction or some other major dysfunction. Once again, health lies in the system's *adaptability* rather than in its *conformation,* as illustrated by the following cases:

> A school requested a psychiatric evaluation of a child with a rare hereditary disease that caused a number of serious handicaps. The mother suffered from the same illness; the child's sibling was spared. The school's attempts to cope with this child were thwarted because the mother refused to carry out the medical component of the child's treatment. The child was therefore forced to experience fully the limitations imposed by her hereditary illness.

> A woman in her mid-twenties brought in her seven-year-old son for evaluation after he had attempted to strangle himself. She described him as "feeling cheated, just like I did, because I have to work all the time." Her developmental history was that of a Cinderella who spent all her time at home doing housework and taking care of her family. Therefore, we can speculate that she projected her sense of being onto her son: i.e., she not only expected, or even *required* him to act cheated but even provided him with opportunities to do so. This was easy for her because of her lifelong pattern of hard work, which cheated her son of *her*!

The most tragic example of this phenomenon is child beating—a repetitious pattern that spans generations. Abusive parents commonly report that having been battered children themselves, they are personally acquainted with the tragic effects of parental violence. They therefore claim to be more motivated than other parents to treat their children with kindness. *This may well be true;* yet they seem almost inexorably drawn into repeating the tragic pattern of brutality.

In summary, then, an examination of the parents's developmental histories may demonstrate that the child's behavior complements the behavior of the parents fairly precisely, and we can infer that this complementarity serves an important function in the family. We should make a special point of searching for multigenerational transmission process (Bowen, 1966) when we see evidence that the parents are encouraging the identified patient's symptomatic behavior.

The parents' developmental histories probably give us our best leverage on the crucial but elusive issue of choice of symptoms: that is, given a level of stress that would lead us to expect breakdown somewhere in the system, why does the family system choose not only a specific symptom *carrier* (the identified patient) but a specific form of symptoms? It has long been known that the child may act out impulses that a parent has long denied and repressed in himself (Johnson, 1949; Szurek, 1942).

A mother sought an evaluation of her son's violent outbursts. On several occasions, however, she gazed calmly at her fingernails as the child attacked the startled examiner. When the examiner asked about her developmental history, he learned that as a child she had been mistreated repeatedly by her older brothers. Therefore, he speculated that she viewed her son's behavior as long-delayed retribution.

A young mother was terrified that her four-year-old son was developing "without any conscience." She described herself as a gentle person who never felt angry or violent, and she was shocked and bewildered when her son attacked and injured other children and displayed no remorse. During his toddlerhood, she had refrained from inhibiting him "because I wanted him to be free." She had spent her own adolescence in virtual seclusion because her parents forbade any social life "if I got any grade below a B, so I just got all Cs and stayed home." She denied being angry at her parents because "I'm a very passive person."

A family sought therapy for their son, who demonstrated extreme passive-aggressive traits. Despite his above-average intelligence, he functioned poorly at school. He consistently won power struggles with his parents and demonstrated elective mutism. At home, he usually did not bother to speak, and when he did speak, his parents had to "strain all the time just to hear him." An almost precise complementarity came to light when we were obtaining the mother's developmental history. She said that in her family, "you had to almost die to get noticed." This was in fact tragically true. After a serious injury in childhood, she suffered excruciating pain, but her parents were oblivious to her complaints and sought medical attention for her only when her life was endangered.

What is the best point during the evaluation to obtain the parents' developmental histories? In some cases, the clinician may prefer to obtain this information early; in others, he may decide to wait until a number of individual or conjoint sessions have taken place. In the latter case, it can be extremely instructive for a parent to observe that the behavioral patterns he so vigorously resents in his own child are faithful copies of those he recalls from his own childhood and that his own behavior as a parent is a faithful copy of parental patterns he vigorously resented as a child. There also may be an opportunity to tie events that occur in conjoint sessions to developmental events: "Now I understand better why you feel so strongly when your child does . . .," for instance. Another interesting option is to elucidate the parental histories gradually in the course of conjoint sessions, linking ongoing process, through affect, to relevent events in the parent's development. For example, "We've talked a lot about the hassles that occur when you ask the children to help with the housework, and I wonder how it was for you, Mrs. Jones, when you had to clean your room when you were at home? How did it go between you and your parents?"

DEVELOPMENT OF THE MARRIAGE AND FAMILY

Because *the family evolves as a unique organism with its own unique characteristics* (see Bowen, 1966; Satir, 1971), it is often useful to ask parents the following questions: "What first attracted you to each other?" and "What holds you together?" Frequently, the marriage has evolved to the point where the original reasons for spending time together are irrelevant. It is often a mind-boggling experience for examiner and married couple alike to deal with this question: "If you met today for the first time, do you think you would fall in love and want to marry each other?" This kind of question is useful, not only because of the information it elicits, but because it teaches us something about the couple's problem-solving style.

Because the family is a system, we are interested in its dynamic properties, which have evolved as a set of rules of adaptation whereby roles (Type II processes) and homeostasis (Type I Processes) are established and maintained. How does the family respond to stress? What maneuvers does it characteristically rely on to maintain homeostasis? How do the identified patient's symptoms relate to this process?

Over time, any organism must maintain a position of balance. If it is too far out of balance, it must do one of two things: change its configuration in response to the stresses that are impinging on it or maintain a constant input of energy to maintain itself as best it can against the unbalancing forces. Families, like all organisms, must solve the problem of maximizing the advantages of their situation while minimizing the amount of energy required to do so. To do so, family members make complex bargains with each other. Some of these bargains are clear and explicit; others are deeply buried and have their roots in the early developmental histories of the parents and other family members. If the family system is built around a large number of hidden bargains, the family may function well under stable conditions and break down under stress. In other words, the family's static properties tell us little about its internal structure, whereas its dynamic properties yield rich information about the family structure and function.

Consider the analogy of a car that is going in a straight line on a smooth road at constant speed. This information establishes only the boundary conditions of the car's functioning. If, on the other hand, we observe the same car on a winding, hilly, bumpy road under a wide variety of weather conditions, we will learn much more and will be able to draw more extensive inferences about the car's structure and function.

In summary, a family's internal structure is often hidden and will become apparent only during a crisis. Therefore, critical data about family roles is best obtained from descriptions of behavior during stressful periods in the family history. Bowen (1966) pointed out that a history of behavior related to crises is extremely useful and that a family in stress can use three means to maintain its balance: (1) one parent may become sick or dysfunctional, (2) marital conflict may occur, or (3) a child may become symptomatic as his parents project onto him aspects of themselves that are overburdened by stress. A special type of stress occurs when certain relationships or situations end. For example death and divorce are unique forms of stress because they necessitate more fundamental rearrangements than do other forms of stress. Therefore, a family's capacity to adapt to crises related to the termination of an important relationship are useful indicators of a mature capacity to grieve loss.

A couple with three children divorced after ten years of marriage. Despite their intentions to maintain a uniform approach to child raising, they used the children to continue their struggle. This inability to resolve their relationship in a creative way, which would have permitted them to continue functioning as parents, revealed the hidden agendas and covert bargains of the previous ten years.

A couple brought their child to the clinic because of his uncontrollable behavior. When the child had reached toddlerhood (any parent who has lived through this stage realizes that the metamorphosis of an adorable infant into a destructive monster is a sizable crisis), the father had resorted to severe punitive measures. This led to a second serious crisis because his wife began to view him as a destructive, harsh, cruel man rather than as the loving, kind individual she had married.

Mr. and Mrs. T came to the clinic in despair. Their difficulties had begun several years earlier when, the night before Mr. T took an important examination, Mrs. T told him she was thinking of leaving him. Although Mr. T informed her that this news distressed him, he spent the night studying and did extremely well on the examination. Because Mr. T had failed to respond as she had hoped, Mrs. T became despondent and concluded that Mr. T was an isolated man who could not be reached, no matter how desperately she tried. In essence, their marriage ended at that point, but they lived together for several more years, maintaining a facade of the successful young marrieds.

FAMILY'S MEDICAL HISTORY

An acute or chronic illness in any family member can represent a serious crisis for the family as a whole—a topic that will be discussed fully in the section on life trauma in Chapter 5. (See also, Anthony & Koupernik, 1973.)

At this point in the evaluation, the clinician should obtain information about familial illnesses such as diabetes and medical or psychological problems such as hyperactivity or reading difficulties. It may also be useful to ask whether the family has a history of problems similar to those of the identified patient. As demonstrated in the following case, this information may be important biologically —in terms of genetic transmission as well as roles—if the family expects the child to turn out "just the way Uncle Harry did."

When ten-year-old Sally, the youngest of four children by her mother's first marriage, was brought to our clinic because she misbehaved at school, she was panicstricken at the sight of the office. The clinician subsequently discovered that Sally's three older siblings had been institutionalized for mental retardation or psychosis. The girl's step-siblings, half-siblings, and acquaintances teased her by saying: "Some day you'll go to a psychiatrist who will lock you up forever." Sally received our diagnosis that she was normal with joy, but her mother responded with a variety of emotions.

In this case, factors involving roles were of overwhelming importance, but an initial glance might have suggested an emphasis on biological factors.

In general, the presence of a serious, chronic illness such as diabetes is an enormous stress that will reduce the amount of energy available to a family for coping with other adaptive needs.

Chapter 5

CHILD'S DEVELOPMENTAL HISTORY

The questions we ask when taking the identified patient's developmental history will immediately reflect our deepest theoretical assumptions. If our primary approach to understanding behavior is biological, we will be interested in a detailed history with regard to pregnancy and delivery, developmental milestones, and so forth. If our primary interest is social, we will direct our questions accordingly. If we view the developing child as a *tabula rasa* or blank slate on which environmental influences impinge to form personality, we have no choice but to infer that psychopathology is the result of a poor environment. Mothers have borne the brunt of this burden, as exemplified by the gruesome term schizophrenogenic mother. (It is only fair to mention that the emphasis on the family—and specifically mothering—as a cause of schizophrenia arose from the hope that schizophrenic patients could be cured through psychotherapy, but the term schizophrenogenic mother has not been without its destructive influence.)

If, on the other hand, we view development as beginning with a biologically unique organism, which will inevitably organize its experience and decide on responses in its
own characteristic way, *starting with syngamy* and proceeding
through its interactions with a complex environment, we
have no need to scapegoat either the child or his environment. Just as length and width are each 100 per cent "responsible" for the total area of a rectangle, so are innate
biological and environmental factors each 100 per cent
"responsible" for the child's development. Therefore, the
objective of this part of the evaluation is an adequate assessment of all significant biological and interactional factors that lead to the evolution of the personality. Table 5.1
compares the interactional structuralist or systems approach with what is probably an unfair and oversimplified
representation of a *tabula rasa* approach.

PREGNANCY

Mother's Physical and Emotional Health

The importance of the mother's physical health is obviously critical. The clinical problem is to select questions
that will yield the greatest payoff for the least effort. The
question "Was your health O.K. during the pregnancy" is
too simple, while a more detailed inquiry can be more
time-consuming than productive. Medications, illnesses of
all kinds, trauma, vaginal bleeding, nutrition, and exposure
to toxins are important, particularly during the first trimes-
ter when fundamental developmental processes occur rapidly. The Collaborative Study of Cerebral Palsy, involving
thousands of infants, has published many papers in this
area, (e.g., Broman, Nichols & Kennedy, 1975; Niswander
& Gordon, 1972; Niswander, Gordon & Drage, 1975) and
Werner, Bierman, and French (1971) and Werner (1976)

Table 5.1   A Comparison of the *Tabula Rasa* and Interactional Structuralist (or Systems) Approaches to Personality Development

Theoretical base and clinical focus	*Simple* Tabula Rasa *model*	*Interactional structuralist or systems approach*
Theoretical base	Causality is parent-to-child only.	Causal relationships exist between all parts of the system. The child and environment participate in actively creating each other.
Meaning of symptoms	Someone has done something bad, either intentionally or unintentionally.	In some cases child-family system has evolved in such a way that someone is in a position to maintain himself at the expense of someone else; his perception of the situation is that he must do so at the present time.
Scapegoating	Inevitably, the conclusion must be: "The parents did it wrong."	Scapegoating is unnecessary: "The family-child system functioned in a way that. . . ."
Objection of evaluation	A diagnosis: i.e., to find the focus of disease so that it can be cured or controlled.	To formulate the relationship between the symptoms and the family's rules of adaptation and explain the current crisis as part of the family's attempt to maintain its balance. To assess the reversibility of symptoms.
Therapist's relationship to parents	Father confessor: "I know that I have done wrong. Please make my child better."	A consultant who assists the family in finding less expensive ways to adapt.

have reported on a long-term longitudinal study of 1,000 children born on the island of Kauai.

The mother's emotional response to prenatal or perinatal trauma can be as significant as the trauma itself. Parental guilt may have contributed to the evolution of a maladaptive distribution of power within the family (see Chapter 8).

Parental Attitudes and Expectations

Because families, not individual women, experience pregnancy, family attitudes and expectations, which in turn are part of a complex social system, are critical to understanding the environment into which the child is born. Anyone who begins a new job goes through a process that is analogous to the one experienced by the newborn child. The formal job description may bear little resemblance to the critical functions to be performed. Although not readily available, information such as the personality of the person who previously held the job, the struggles that evolved within that situation, and the organization's hopes that the new employee will solve the problem or prove someone's point may have a tremendous impact on the new employee's experience. In other words, the new employee steps into not only a formal job description but a complex belief structure. The same is true of the newborn.

Ideally, the environment responds in a loving, supportive way to any child, regardless of his sex, temperament, and the like. This ideal, of course, does not occur in the real world, and couples have many motivations for pregnancy. Clinically, the question is "What did you want the child to do *for* you?" If the parents had fairly specific expectations about the child's curative properties for the family and if these expectations have not been fulfilled, the parents have no option but to feel angry and disappointed and may well resent the child's demands on them. Their attitude can then easily become: "You have not done for us what we wanted. After all we've done for you, why should we take care of you?" When the child is adopted, these issues can be even more intense and complicated. The following cases illustrate the high-risk situations that can develop as a result of parental expectations and attitudes:

> After delivering her twelfth child—a boy—a middle-aged woman commented in a resigned and depressed tone: "Oh, I wanted another girl; I got ten boys at home already!" It was tragically obvious in this case that the child's development was in severe jeopardy from the beginning.

> The mother of the identified patient was the youngest of three sisters. She had always viewed herself as competing unsuccessfully with the older two, both of whom had adjusted admirably to motherhood and had produced admirable children. Therefore, it was obvious that extreme demands would be placed on any child born into this family, regardless of its sex, temperament, or other factors. But a child of the "wrong" sex and a difficult temperament would help to create an especially high-risk situation.

DELIVERY

Because most women are now conscious during delivery, they can provide useful information about the child's health at birth. For instance, does the mother recall whether the physician expressed any special concern about the child, was the child placed in an incubator after birth, and so forth. The newborn child is competent to withstand trauma and, except in extreme cases of neonatal morbidity, there is no strong correlation between the baby's condition at birth and his subsequent level of functioning (Wolff, 1967). However, if the child fails to cry immediately or must be put in an incubator, for instance, these factors may have not only biological implications but a profound and persistent impact on the child-family system.

Eight-year-old Mary wielded an extraordinary amount of power over her parents by resorting to aggressive behavior during meals. Any time she indicated she would not eat, her parents became extremely anxious. At birth Mary had weighed four pounds, ten ounces and had gained weight slowly as an infant, although her general health was good. Her conscientious mother, guilt-ridden about the baby's small size, became so anxious about the issue of feeding that the entire child-family system was massively distorted.

INFANCY

Health

If the child's pattern of growth is normal, the chance of a significant metabolic disorder is small; however, a lag in growth may be related to one of many factors. Standard curves for height, weight, and head circumference are available and should be used in every workup.

Temperamental Type

Although it is often difficult, when taking a child's history, to delineate his temperamental traits clearly, the clinician should be able to obtain a general impression of the child's temperamental type (easy, slow to warm up, or difficult)—or the mother's memory of it—by asking the mother the kinds of questions listed in Table 5.2. The representative answers contained in the table and the problems described in the following case indicate that it is not difficult to discover which temperamental traits cause stress or are adaptive in the child-parent system:

> Mrs. R's difficulties with her fourth baby could be traced to early mother-child interactions that were extremely distressing to her. The child reacted intensely to stimuli and exhibited a low degree of rhythmicity. For example, his

Table 5.2 Sample Questions and Answers That Will Reveal A Child's Temperamental Traits

Trait	Typical Question	Typical Parental Description
Activity level	As an infant, did the child kick off his blankets at night? Did he move around in his crib a lot? Has he always been active? Did you feel a lot of activity before he was born?	He moved all around, even when he was asleep. He was always on the go. He never was still even as a baby; he wiggled all the time. (high activity level.)
Rhythmicity	Did the child eat, sleep, and have bowel movements pretty much on a predictable schedule? Was it easy to develop a good feeding schedule?	I could never tell when he'd want to be fed; sometimes every two hours, then every six, then two again. He has always gone to bed at different times. (Low degree of rhythmicity.)
Approach/withdrawal	Does the child tend to respond to a new situation by moving into it? Does he tend to hang back in response to a new situation? As a baby, did he like new foods?	He always goes right after new things (approach). He tends to hang back in a strange situation (withdrawal).
′ Adaptability	Does the child tolerate change easily? Does he respond easily to suggestions? Does he tend to respond to discipline by changing his behavior in the direction you want? Do strange situations seem to disturb him (this reaction should be differentiated from withdrawal, the child is not upset but simply responds to novelty by "hanging back").	He has always been comfortable in new situations. Changes in the environment, or what we expect, etc. doesn't seem to upset him.

Table 5.2 (continued)

Trait	Typical Question	Typical Parental Description
Intensity of reactions	Does the child tend to react full scale whether laughing or crying? When he was a baby, did he scream about a wet diaper or just complain? Does it seem that everything, good and bad, is a big deal?	He just doesn't have a mid-range. If something strikes him funny, he screams with laughter. If he's even a little hurt, he howls at the top of his lungs. (Intense reactions).
Quality of mood	Is he generally cheerful? Does he tend to be irritable and fussy?	He's always been a happy, cheerful baby (positive mood). He was colicky as a baby and he's usually whiney and ornery (negative mood).
Persistence attention span	Does the child stick to a task? Does he work for long periods of time on one thing?	Once he started something, he would stick to it no matter what. He didn't get tired of playing with the same toy for a long time. (High persistence attention span).
Distractibility	Is the child easily pulled away from something he is doing?	Any noise, or somebody entering the room was enough to get his attention away from a toy or even food. (High degree of distractibility).
Threshold to stimuli	Would you describe your child as a hair-trigger kid? Does it take much to set him off, one way or another?	Anything at all was enough to get a reaction: a whisper was as good as a shout. (Low Threshold).

exasperated mother reported that one day he would refuse to eat at six o'clock and would scream for a bottle at ten. The next day he would eat hungrily at six o'clock and sleep soundly throughout the night. On the third day he would eat small meals periodically throughout the night. Her other children had displayed only moderately intense reactions and a high degree of rhythmicity. Therefore, it is easy to understand why the fourth child's temperament led to severe problems of self-esteem in both mother and child. One can picture the distress of both as Mrs. R asked him again and again: "Why can't you be like your brothers and sisters?" Lacking the concept of temperamental type, Mrs. R was faced with a difficult set of options: she was a bad mother, the child willfully chose to be difficult, or she was being punished for her sins.

Although Mrs. R struggled to relate to all her children the same way, she found that this was impossible. As a result, relatives, neighbors, and her three older children criticized her for giving the fourth child special favors. Inevitably, this child became the scapegoat for all the family's difficulties. Mrs. R's attempts to maintain her self-esteem in the face of this constant pounding caused him to develop severe symptoms at an early age, which further justified the evolving myth of "bad child."

Although clinicians tend to focus on difficult cases, it should be noted that most child-family systems evolve in a positive, synergistic way: i.e., the child's temperament interacts with the family structure in a manner that brings joy to all. Thus, in a healthy child-family system, the whole becomes greater than the sum of its parts.

It is often clinically useful to introduce parents to the concept of temperamental type and point out that a difficult child will be a challenge to any parents in any environment. Many parents experience an immediate and dramatic decrease in anxiety and guilt when they realize that their child's difficult behavior is not necessarily the result of bad parenting!

After a reasonable amount of experience, the clinician may be able to obtain a temperamental profile with relative ease and without traumatizing the parents.

Early Parent-child Interactions

It is often impossible to assess the general direction of the evolution of the parent-child system by asking a few questions about the first interactions between the parents and child. In general, the parent-child system should operate in terms of simple feedback principles which generate interaction that is gratifying to both parties. For example, the child cries, indicating distress; the parent decodes this signal correctly and carries out appropriate measures such as changing his diaper, feeding him, or bouncing him gently. If the parent-child system is malfunctioning, the parent or child will ignore or misread the signals. Because any complex system can become imbalanced and break down at any point, it is useful to obtain some idea of the specific locus of the difficulty. Are the frequency and intensity of the child's distress signals too high? Is the parent's capacity to respond appropriately inadequate? Is the child unable to inform his parents adequately that he has been well cared for? For example:

Mrs. L requested an evaluation of John because he was "unmanageable." Mrs. L was a demanding person who set high standards for herself and then drove herself unmercifully to meet them. Her mother lived in the same neighborhood and constantly added fuel to Mrs. L's intrapsychic fire by criticizing her incessantly. When asked about the initial mother-child interactions, Mrs. L stated: "It was just terrible. I rang the buzzer for the nurse every few minutes because something was always wrong." The interactions between this mother and child were gratifying to neither, and Mr. L could provide no assistance. Mrs. L was frantic because John constantly assaulted her self-esteem rather than gratifying her wish to be a perfect mother. Mrs. L's relationship to her own mother, of course, was a severe complication.

Mrs X, whose own developmental history had been chaotic, had been unable to respond to the appropriate cries of her infant son, Danny. She had interpreted his cries to mean that she was a bad mother, which embarrassed her in the presence of numerous relatives who lived in the same apartment building. Therefore, she responded to his cries by bellowing: "Danny, you be a good boy and be quiet!" As he grew older, Danny displayed a pathetic, depressed appearance. Had he been of a different temperament, physical abuse might well have occurred.

A mother who considered herself useless described her ten-year-old daughter, Anne, as "living in her own dream world." During Anne's infancy, her mother had interpreted happy behavior to mean that Anne did not need her; if Anne cried or was unhappy, her mother knew she was needed. Therefore, the rules of this mother-child system required Anne to be miserable. The child resolved this dilemma by withdrawing into her own fantasy life.

A few questions about early mother-child interactions will yield critical information about how the mother-child system evolved, how gratifying it is, and what problem-solving maneuvers the family and child use to cope with difficulties. The rigorous clinician will consider these events formally in terms of the family's rules of adaptation. For example, who first recognized that the system was not functioning properly? Who took responsibility for maintaining balance? How did these patterns evolve? Occasionally, family patterns that were observable as early as the first few feedings will remain stable throughout a child's development.

Shifts in Parental Attitudes

Earlier, I mentioned the importance of the parents' fantasies about what the new baby would be like. The ability to adapt to a new reality is the *sine qua non* of a healthy system. Thus, the parents' capacity to adapt to the unpredictable reality of their new baby yields critical information about their adaptability as individuals and as a family. For instance, if a couple want a girl but have a boy, the obvious adaptive reaction is to accept the child as what he is. A maladaptive response would be to insist that the child gratify his parents' expectations.

Fundamentally, what we are talking about here is the family's capacity to grieve the loss of something that is an important part of their reference system, whether in reality or in fantasy. In other words, we want to know whether the family system is capable of changing the reference system with respect to which it functions. If these Type II changes cannot be carried out, the parents have no choice but to rely on Type I processes: i.e., to force the child to accommodate to their expectations so that they can assimilate him into the existing family structure. Clearly, the child's sex and temperament will determine how difficult this process will be for everyone concerned.

DEVELOPMENTAL LANDMARKS

Physical Growth

A description of developmental landmarks has traditionally been a core component of evaluation. Geselle and Amatruda (1947) have summarized a wealth of developmental data, and the Denver Developmental Scale developed by Frankenburg and Dodds (1967) provides a rough but useful means of assessing a child's level of development. In the case of a primarily biological problem, these data are critically important.

Parents' perceptions of and reactions to an infant's rate and pattern of development are always important, regardless of the child's actual developmental course or the

unreliability of the parents' recollections about his development. Because how the parents respond to their past
perceptions of the child's developmental course is often
more useful for our purposes than scientifically reliable
developmental data would be, major milestones in the
child's development should be noted. But if deviations are
not apparent to a reasonably skilled observer, the clinician
must decide whether to pursue the matter in greater detail
or move on to another topic.

Psychological Growth

Although norms for children's cognitive and interpersonal
development are far less clear than are norms for their
physical development, it is important to determine whether
the parents perceived the child as developing normally and
at a normal rate.

When attempting to assess cognitive development and
functioning, the clinician may find that contacting the
school is adequate. A more extensive assessment, of
course, is the province of the psychologist. Anastasi's work
in this area (1968) is central, and Buros (1970) has com-
piled a comprehensive summary of all the instruments
available for making such an assessment. In addition, the
complex issues involved in cognitive development have
been explored by a number of authors (see, for example,
Flavell, 1963; Kohlberg, 1968; Lenneberg, 1969; Mussen,
1970; Santostefano, 1969).

The normal child's affective and interpersonal development progresses through the following stages: the first
social smiles of infancy, delight with the "peek-a-boo"
game, anxiety when approached by strangers, "autistic"
play, parallel play, social play, "best-buddy" phase, competitive games, and peer-group interaction. Serious deviations from this normal chain of development may be
apparent as early as the first feeding if the child is autistic,

develop more insidiously in the schizoid child, or take a wide variety of forms in the depressed child.

EVOLUTION OF PERSONALITY

As mentioned in Chapter 2, temperamental type can be conceptualized as the biological precursor of personality. In operational terms, temperamental type indicates the probability that the child will demonstrate certain patterns of response and activity throughout life. Personality can be defined in similar terms (Hall & Lindzey, 1970). Thus personality evolves from temperament as the child structures his perception of the world through his interactions with it.

Taking a developmental history provides an excellent opportunity for sensitive clinical interviewing. The task requires a knowledge of normal development and an ability to follow indications of abnormal processes. Overall, the sense that caring for and interacting with the child was satisfying and often fun for the parents is central. Remember that a child (and the child-family system) is "born" many times; the tasks of infancy bear little resemblance to those of latency. The development of stranger anxiety late in the first year, or mobility a few months later, may force a significant rearrangement in the family.

The printed page can only hope to provide the bare bones. Skill requires practice. In Table 5.3 I have tried to summarize the essential processes of each stage.

INTERACTIONAL FACTORS:
EVOLUTION OF ROLE AND SELF-IMAGE

Interactions with Family

The family's specific strengths will determine the developmental stages of childhood that can be supported and nur-

Table 5.3 Questions Designed to Elicit Information About the Child's Psychosocial-Psychosexual Development[a]

Stage	Sample Questions
I. basic trust versus basic mistrust	Did you enjoy taking care of the baby? Did the baby feed well and thrive? How did weaning go? How did you and the baby decide when it should eat? Did the baby cuddle?
II. autonomy versus shame and doubt	Did you move your belongings to protect them from your toddlers, or did you insist that the child learn to leave things alone? How did you handle temper tantrums? How did toilet training occur? How did you feel about the insistent "No's" of the toddler? What kind of discipline did you use when this became necessary? How did the child respond?
III. Preschool: initiative versus guilt	Did the child develop interests outside the home? Was there excessive jealousy about the attachment between you and your spouse? Did the child seem eager to develop and enjoy his rapidly expanding abilities? Did he insist on sleeping with you? If so, did you and your spouse agree about how this should be handled?
IV. Grade school: industry versus inferiority	How did the child's first years of school go? Did he find satisfaction in doing his school work? How did the family respond when he brought school work home? Did the child enjoy hobbies, making things and so on.
V. Adolescence: identity versus role confusion	Do you have a good sense of yourself and the way you relate to your friends, mate, and career?

[a]Based on Erikson's Eight Ages of Man (1950).

tured comfortably. Unbalanced areas will force the family to look for a balancing influence. If the child's temperament or other characteristics seem appropriate, the family is likely to use him as a balancing influence, as demonstrated in the following examples:

> In a family of four children, one child demonstrated a high activity level, positive mood, moderate adaptability, and a tendency to withdraw when confronted with new situations. Another exhibited a positive mood, a high degree of activity and adaptability, and a tendency to approach novel situations willingly. The family's needs were such that the shy child played a Cinderella role, staying home and helping with the chores, and so forth. The sibling, who met the family's requirements for a highly successful and visible family member, was involved in many school activities. Although the roles of these children initially arose because of complex interaction between their temperamental types and the family's needs and strengths, certain aspects of these roles were eventually defined as symptoms by both children.

> One young couple, who were suffering severe marital strife and whose ability to express anger toward each other was limited, had an extremely active child with a low reaction threshold, high activity level, low rhythmicity, and a tendency to approach new situations willingly. Each parent began using this difficult and challenging child as a messenger of anger to the other. Their marriage thus obtained support where it was most deficient. (This warfare configuration will be described fully in Chapter 8.) Unfortunately, this pattern violated the rule that there is no free lunch.

Other Interactions

Do the child's interactions at school, with peers, and so on indicate his family provides a stable base as he moves progressively into the world and uses the resources of the social system? Can the child develop a variety of coping maneuvers and use them in a flexible, adaptive way? These questions are closely related to the concept of differentiation and to the temperamental traits of adaptability, approach, and mood.

HISTORY OF LIFE TRAUMA.　How the family evolves as a social system and the role of crises in this process were discussed earlier. Similarly, crises in an individual's life may lead to adaptation (an improved ability to cope) or to regression (a permanently weakened state). According to Menninger (1962), information about stresses can be summarized most easily in the form of a chart. The chart might include: (1) the timing and nature of traumatic events, (2) the patient's age and major resources available at the time, (3) the qualitative nature of his reactions to the trauma, (4) the nature of his coping maneuvers and rate of recovery, and (5) any evidence that after the trauma, he was able to cope better with stress, acquired permanent symptoms, never regained his earlier level of functioning, or was less capable of handling stress.

> When John was six years old, his aunt told him that he was not his father's son but the child of his mother's first husband. In other words, he was "not really part of the family." At the time, John lived with his mother, two siblings, and a group of relatives in the relatives' home while his step-father was in the army. Shortly after, he became morose, irritable, and depressed. According to his mother, "John's been crabby off and on ever since." (He had always been a cheerful child before.) He began sleepwalking and was found in odd places in the morning. Although he seemed to respond well to play therapy with a male therapist over a period of a year, he reverted to his original symptoms immediately when the therapist left the agency.

> A four-year-old girl was hospitalized with a salmonella infection and was isolated for several weeks. Since the family dog she loved deeply was the primary carrier, it was destroyed in her absence. This led to a variety of symptomatic behav-

iors. Play therapy led to a positive resolution of the problem: the girl asked for, received, and enjoyed another dog.

Coddington (1972 a and b) ranked a variety of life events according to their traumatic effect on children of different ages. Thus it is possible to estimate, in rough, quantitative terms, the number of life change units that have accumulated over the previous year.

Note that the identified patient's medical history is included twice in section IV of the outline, once under "Specific Interactional Factors" and again under "Medical History." This dual listing reflects my bias about the importance of understanding an illness in terms of the context in which it occurs and, in particular, the impact it has on the family belief system. At all times, but especially during a crisis, a child will carefully observe his parents for the *meaning* of events.

Piaget's concept of preoperational thought is useful in this context, as demonstrated by the following case:

Jerry, age three, seemed unable to tolerate separation from his mother. He had been hospitalized eight times before he was 14 months old and his fear of separation had increased with each hospitalization. By the time he was three, he was alternately panic-stricken and assaultive when taken to nursery school. During the course of play therapy, it became evident that he had magically linked his illnesses and associated events with the progressive deterioration which had simultaneously occurred in his family. His repeated illnesses had in fact become a convenient scapegoat for other family difficulties, and the notion that he was responsible for those difficulties was communicated to him in various ways. The egocentrism and magical causality that are characteristic of children his age would make him far more vulnerable to this process than would be the case if his cognitive structure permitted him to see that his behavior had not, in fact, been the cause of the family's difficulties. Furthermore, centration (the inability to see a complex process as composed of several independent variables) would make it impossible to differentiate between the consequences of his behavior, thoughts, and illness.

MEDICAL HISTORY

Earlier, I discussed the importance of maternal health during pregnancy, perinatal hazards, and health during infancy. Here, we are concerned with extraordinary illness of any kind, past or current medications, allergies, trauma, hospitalizations, special diet, exposure to toxins, and the like. The role that allergies play in behavioral disorders in children is currently the subject of active debate. Repeated fractures or lacerations, for example, may reflect depression, expressed as accident proneness or outright self-destructive behavior. We are just beginning to appreciate the role of depression in self-destructive behavior in children (For a detailed discussion about the role of family illness in the depression and suicide attempt of a seven-year-old boy, see French & Steward, 1975.) Here as elsewhere, illness may be important for a variety of reasons at both the biological and role levels (Szurek, 1942).

Brief inquiries can be made, possibly while obtaining data for the family tree, about the presence of (1) serious, chronic illnesses in the family, (2) familial illnesses such as diabetes, (3) emotional or psychiatric disorders (a specific question frequently yields a positive finding; families rarely volunteer the information), and (4) disorders that resemble those of the identified patient.

Chapter 6

CLINICAL OBSERVATIONS

Clinical observations should ideally take place in so relaxed and comfortable a manner that the patient and family have no sense of being interviewed. The clinician should learn to obtain as much information as possible from each perspective and drop any avenue of approach that ceases to be productive. "Personal" questions need rarely be asked; inferences of great import can be made from readily available data. This chapter seeks to describe a number of different observational perspectives.

FAMILY'S BEHAVIOR IN THE WAITING ROOM

Observing the child and his family in the waiting room is an excellent way to obtain uncontaminated data. It is usually possible to identify the family, before they have an opportunity to identify you, by walking through the waiting room once or twice to observe the behavior of individual family members and how members interact with one another. Frequently, these initial patterns of interaction will remain constant throughout a number of sessions.

> A middle-aged woman and her preadolescent son were evaluated because of the son's school failure. While in the waiting room, mother and son sat close together, reading intently. The posture of each was virtually identical in every detail. Subsequent work confirmed this "carbon-copy" relationship between the two in virtually all areas of their lives. Gradually, the two began to adopt their own sitting positions in the waiting room, and this behavior faithfully forecast what would occur in the day's session.

> A young woman who described her son, Tim, as "a difficult child who never minds anything I say" was observed in the waiting room. Tim stood in front of the candy machine loudly demanding a candy bar. His mother insisted repeatedly that she would not give him one, but his demands only intensified with her repeated denials. Finally, in an exasperated tone, she said: "Oh, all right, but be sure to put it in your pocket until we're through seeing the doctor." When the candy bar was placed in his hands, Tim quieted down and immediately began removing the wrapper. A similar argument ensued about eating the candy bar. This pattern, which effectively reinforced Tim's obnoxious behavior, permeated every facet of their interaction.

CHILD'S BEHAVIOR IN THE OFFICE OR PLAYROOM

The clinical interview with the identified patient has been discussed by many authors (e.g., Chess, 1969; Goodman & Sours, 1967; Simmons, 1969). Therefore, I will simply point out that if the patient is an adolescent, it is essential to clarify, with the parents as well as the patient, the nature of the working alliance and what will be shared with whom under what circumstances. I prefer to see an adolescent alone first and subsequently see him together with all other available family members.

The nuances of establishing rapport with smaller children are learned best through observation, experience, and instinct. The objective of this section is to outline clinical tools that require a minimum amount of intervention on the clinician's part. The child's reaction when separated from his parents and his general appearance and behavior are obvious. Observations in the office occasionally lead to questions about specific temperamental traits. More active inquiries may be required to learn about the child's problem-solving abilities and style, although fortuitous observations often provide useful leads.

SEPARATION FROM PARENTS.   How a child behaves when left alone with the clinician provides useful information about many aspects of functioning including temperament, mastery of appropriate psychosexual stages—especially Stage I (basic trust versus basic mistrust) and Stage II (autonomy versus shame and doubt)—and the overall parent-child system. Sometimes the parent's separation anxiety is greater than the child's. As shown in the following examples, these data are particularly useful because they are often relatively uncontaminated and occur fairly naturally and spontaneously.

> *Approach versus withdrawal.* A six-year-old described by the school as impossibly disruptive spent only a few minutes in the waiting room before asking his mother which office belonged to the doctor he would see. When she pointed out my office from the waiting room, he walked across the room and knocked on my door, announcing "I am your four o'clock patient." His developmental history confirmed that he always responded to novelty with approach.

> *Basic trust versus mistrust.* The developmental history of, the three-year-old described in Chapter 5, who had been hospitalized eight times during the first 14 months of life, would

obviously predispose him to problems related to Stage I issues. In the office, he cried and clung to his mother when she got up to leave. She promised to wait for him "right outside the door," and after more protests, he finally agreed. But shortly after she left, he ran to the door, opened it, and discovered that she had returned to the waiting room. He ran to her and refused to come into my office again.

Autonomy versus shame and doubt. When I asked the mother of a five-year-old to leave so that he and I could talk together, he jumped up, ran to the door, and blocked her exit. She quietly asked him to move, but he yelled "No" and began kicking at her as she tried to approach the door. She responded by pleading with him to be reasonable.

Parent-child interaction. A mother requested an evaluation of her adolescent son Tom because he was destructive at home. Over the telephone she said Tom was so difficult that she was convinced that one of them would have to leave home soon unless drastic changes were made. In the waiting room, Tom slept on the couch. His mother said he had a headache and she hated to disturb him, but when I asked her to, she did so. As Tom stood up, she put her arm around him; he did not reciprocate this gesture. As he turned to enter my office, she kept her hands on his shoulders as long as she could and then, as he walked away, stood with her arms extended toward him. This marked ambivalence, characterized by hostility and overprotection, was typical of their relationship.

Separation from parents is often a problem for young children. Although one occasionally resorts to picking up a child, carrying him screaming into the office, and sitting in front of the door while he frantically attempts to return to his parent, it would be difficult to view this as the method of choice. In the case of a young child, I prefer to see parent and child together initially and later ask the parent to leave. If I am especially interested in testing the child's tendency to experience abandonment anxiety, I may, after some time has elapsed, leave him alone in the office. This is accomplished most gracefully when he is drawing or playing.

A ten-year-old with an air of bravado and a swaggering tough-guy manner became somewhat uneasy when his mother left him in my office. While he was working on a drawing, I said I would have to leave the office for a few minutes; during this time he could work undisturbed. He did not look up from his drawing, but I was no more than ten feet down the hallway when he dashed out looking for me. Although I assured him I would not be gone long, he said he preferred to accompany me on my errand.

Appearance, Behavior, and Attitude

A few descriptive sentences will usually provide a clear picture of the patient, as shown in these brief examples:

Fifteen-year-old Eddie "bopped" into the office, bounced into a chair, jauntily lit a cigarette, and demanded an ashtray. He was dressed in the latest "mod" style. After looking directly at the clinician for a few moments, he commented: "Well, you look about as crazy as the last few shrinks they've sent me to."

Dave, age five, sat quietly, looking straight ahead. He answered questions quickly and nervously. When asked about his parents' conflicts, he sobbed uncontrollably for several minutes.

Temperamental Type

In addition to using the parents' descriptions of the identified patient's temperament, I also make my own assessment, particularly by looking for traits that are relevant to the chief complaint and presenting problems. Chess (1969) urged clinicians to seek the parents' assessment of the child's temperamental type in infancy and at six years of age and to make an additional assessment based on his own observations of the child behavior. It is convenient to collect these data on a form such as the one shown in the Appendix.

Problem-solving Style

One can approach this topic with varying degrees of structure. An open approach, such as providing the child with free access to toys, may demonstrate how he imposes structure. From such data, it is possible to draw inferences concerning the nature of his internal structure. Specific tasks, challenges, or stimuli, on the other hand, can be used to test specific areas of functioning or to explore the child's capacity to handle conflict.

It is possible to get some idea about the child's cognitive processes by asking him for projective material related to drawings or stories, by observing him at play, and so forth:

> Nine-year-old Danny was hostile and angry when his parents separated. In the office, however, he was usually cooperative and preferred to talk about baseball. He described his feelings about his parents' separation as follows: "It's like you're playing the World Series and the score is three to three, and you're playing the last game, and the game is three to nothing and your team is losing and it's two strikes and three balls and there's three men on base and you're up to bat." Danny's egocentric view of the situation is obvious. Thus one might evaluate his feelings in terms of magical causality: i.e., he felt responsible for his parent's marital difficulties. With his permission, I raised this issue later in a session that included his parents.

It is often useful, when attempting to assess an individual's (or family's) interpersonal problem-solving style, to confront him with moderate stress. The clinical task, of course, is to present a stress that, although not traumatic, will test the individual's capacity to reestablish a balance after a noticeable jolt. For example, I mentioned earlier that I sometimes ask couples: "If you met today for the first time, would you have any interest in each other?" Or, in a situation where I am dealing with an apparently healthy and normal child and am finding it difficult to substantiate a chief complaint about his unruliness at home, I may intentionally upset the child by "accidentally" knocking over a tower of blocks he has carefully constructed.

Other more specific tasks can be presented to the child in an attempt to relate his coping maneuvers directly to specific temperamental traits or to dynamic material. For example, the traits of distractibility and persistence/attention span, which are critically important in school, can be observed by walking noisily in and out of the office, banging desk drawers, and so on while the child is drawing. As the following case illustrates, a child's problem-solving style may raise questions about areas of conflict and about temperamental traits:

A young mother asked us to evaluate five-year-old Wendy because of the child's clinging, dependent behavior. While the family was in the waiting room, I noticed that Wendy, her mother, and the mother's older sister were poring intently over the form that is given routinely to new patients. The aunt then took Wendy to the restroom. As the child emerged from the restroom, she ran to her mother with open arms, exclaimed "MOTHER!" and leaped happily into her mother's arms; the two fondly hugged each other as though they had been separated longer than a few minutes. In the playroom, I tried to assess the child's fantasies about the absence of mother. To do so, I used the playhouse, saying "Here is the mother—she is going for a long trip." I then moved the mother to a distant point behind some obstacles. Wendy pursued the "lost" mother by car and airplane and attacked me physically when I got in her way. Because of her behavior, I decided to consider in detail the child's temperamental traits of persistence and attention span; her intelligence; her developmental history, paying special attention to difficulties involving basic trust versus mistrust and autonomy versus shame and doubt; and the possibility that she filled a special role in the family.

Behavior During Interviews

Among the tools used to "interview" a child, unstructured play—although time consuming—is most projective and therefore least contaminated by the clinician's preconceptions.

PLAY.   A diagnostic play session can be treated as a projective test by inviting the child to use any toys he wishes. The examiner can then carefully pursue certain themes and gain insights into the nature of the child's fantasy structure, cognitive and interactional styles, and the like. Clinicians who are bored with playroom material would find the same material exciting and dramatic if it was presented by an adult as a dream. Therefore, if you find you are bored in the playroom, remember that the child is sharing with you a part of his fantasy structure, just as an adult does when reporting a dream. And it is as important to minimize one's projections and resultant distortions of play material as it is when handling an adult patient's dream. The obvious difference in the two situations is that it is essential to interact with the child's play material in some way. One way is to follow the child's instructions carefully: for example, if the child chooses puppets, insist that *he* supply most of the dialogue that takes place between them. This will maximize his projections.

DRAWINGS.   Drawing can be highly projective ("draw anything you like") or specifically structured ("please draw a picture of your family with everyone doing something").

Most clinicians ask children to do a drawing of a person as a standard projective test. I usually offer a child color crayons, although occasionally one will ask for a pen or pencil. I try to obtain three drawings: one of anything the child wishes to draw, one of a person, and one of the entire family.

Because drawings tend to be overinterpreted, the clinician must draw inferences from them with great care. As shown in the following example, the traditional Draw-a-Person test (Harris, 1964) can be used as a reference point for future comparisons and often provides interesting leads.

> A mother who described her seven-year-old son as "too much for me to handle" had been divorced for five years and was seriously depressed. Her son, on the other hand, seemed asymptomatic. The family lived a short distance from the mother's parents, successful professionals who had been married for more than twenty years and had suffered no obvious, serious crises. The boy's drawing of a person was of a large, strong looking man. When the therapist asked who the man was, the child paused for a moment and then said: "Well, I am not sure. I think it is either me or my grandfather."

It is easy to pursue a child's fantasies about the figure he has drawn simply by asking "What kind of a person is she? Does she have any friends?" and so forth. Occasionally, it is useful to ask a child to tell a story about the person in the drawing. In the context of a drawing of the family, it is useful to ask the child to drawing each member engaged in a characteristic activity (a technique called the Kinetic Family Drawing, Burns & Kaufman, 1970).

> A five-year-old made the following comments as he drew members of his family: "Here is my dad, workin' on the car like he does all the time. Here's me, handing him a wrench, but he doesn't see me cause he's looking at the engine of the car. He can't hear me either because the engine is running. Here's my little sister, buggin' me. If she doesn't shut up, I going to hit her with the wrench. And here's my mom, yellin' at my dad. But he doesn't hear her either.

It is astonishing when a withdrawn and reticent child who insists that things are fine at home suddenly blossoms forth with this kind of material. Things are "fine" if they are "normal"; the drawing helps us understand the child's definition of normality. The literature abounds with examples of this type, which challenge the clinician to avoid overprojection. Inferences cannot be safely drawn unless there is at least a reasonable degree of consistency between independent observations.

WISHES AND FANTASIES.   Those who seek a formulation of behavior based on inferred preconscious and unconscious processes must obtain maximally projective, minimally contaminated material provided by stories, wishes, and fantasies. Many clinicians ask children to describe what they would do with three magic wishes. According to Gardner (1972), however, five wishes are more useful since the first three tend be ordinary, while the last two are more projective. Children will often report dreams if asked. Strong and recurrent dreams are especially valuable, of course.

In the context of gaining information about the child's fantasy structure, Gardner's storytelling technique (1971) merits special mention. This technique calls for a tape recorder—preferably of the cassette type so that the child's cassette can be used over a number of sessions. The child is asked to tell a brand new story to an imaginary audience. (Gardner described this technique as producing a dream on demand.)

This technique, like all other clinical techniques, is subject to misuse by both patient and therapist, but it is gratifying when children who are extremely guarded present material to the tape recorder in a therapist's presence. When the story is played back to the patient, his reactions can be as illuminating as those of an adult patient who has been asked to describe the most striking aspect of his dream. Of course, Gardner used this technique not only as an evaluative tool but as a therapeutic one, and his book is filled with clinical material about its use. In essence, it includes observing the child's conflict and then retelling the story with a healthier resolution of the conflict.

I am more comfortable with a somewhat conservative version of Gardner's technique. Rather than retell the entire story myself, I say: "That's a very interesting story.

Let's you and I together tell it over again." I then repeat the first few lines of the story and stop at a specific point, giving the child the opportunity to restructure the material. It is exciting when the youngster eagerly interrupts to carry the story to a new conclusion, using a healthier and more adaptive set of coping mechanisms than he did in the first version.

One valuable aspect of Gardner's technique is that when the story is played back to the child, the clinician will discover something about the child's capacity to relate to and work with the material—some of which is likely to be emotionally loaded.

When dealing with a frightened child, the therapist must be deft or the child may become uneasy about presenting fantasy material. For example, a slender preadolescent girl with a variety of gastrointestinal problems agreed, somewhat reluctantly, to tell the following story to the recorder:

> There were two shepherds. These shepherds had a large flock of sheep but noticed that seven of the sheep were missing. When they went to look for them, they found two foxes and one sheep. They opened the foxes' mouths and pulled out the six sheep which the foxes had swallowed.

Were these sheep O.K.?
Yes, they were O.K.
What happened then?
Well, the two shepherds killed the two foxes and ate them.

After hearing the story, the girl refused to tell any more stories to the tape recorder for a long time.

VIEW OF THE EVALUATION.   Many mothers tell a child he is going to see a doctor. Thus children are often bewildered by a visit to a doctor's office where there are toys rather than white coats, examining tables, and needles. As shown in the following examples, the child's view of the evaluation provides useful insights into his relationship with his parents as well as his attitude about his symptomatic behavior.

> An eight-year-old was brought in for an evaluation because of his lying, violence, and fire-setting. He sat in my office somewhat glumly. When I asked "Did you mind coming in?" the youngster merely nodded. But when I asked "Were you afraid you'd get a shot?" replied: "Oh no. I don't mind getting shots, but talking about your family can be pretty scary." Two days after this evaluation, the boy was sent to live permanently with a distant relative.

> Ten-year-old Sandy, described by the school as hyperactive, came from a home where the parents quarreled constantly. One subject of their arguments was the value of psychiatric intervention. When asked how he felt about seeing a psychiatrist, Sandy said: "Well, I think it is a lousy idea. All psychiatrists ever do is just lock people up and put electricity in their heads so they have bad convulsions and get sick. Then they put them away forever." Obviously, it was difficult for Sandy to be cooperative, and a conflict between his parents subsequently emerged as one of the most important factors in the overall picture.

Thought Processes and Language Structure

The therapist should quote a child's idiosyncratic language in the chart verbatim rather than simply label it as psychotic or loosely associated.

> A five-year-old whose parents had long been concerned about her development had been labeled with a variety of serious diagnoses. When the therapist asked her how she felt about an incident that occurred during the session, she replied: "Happy! Happy! Birthday, happy!" and then sang "Happy Birthday to you, Happy birthday to you. . . ." This performance demonstrated the child's ability to identify a

specific affect and communicate it to another person by means of an association that was clearly relevant. In other words, although her thought processes were obviously idiosyncratic, she also had some good communication skills.

It is far more useful to seek a detailed understanding of the precise nature of the child's abnormality (e.g., does he always "spiral off" into his first association to an affect? Does he express his first association in all situations?) than to label it as schizophrenic or autistic.

The parents of an eight-year-old, who had been diagnosed as schizophrenic, autistic, and mentally retarded, requested a complete workup and diagnosis. In the playroom, she seemed unable to answer the simplest questions and instead repeated the last few words of the therapist's questions. She began playing with a teddy bear and toy telephone. She held the receiver to the teddy bear's ear, then handed it to the therapist, and looking directly at him said: "Here, the teddy bear wants to talk to you." This one statement demonstrated the child's ability to see the relationship between herself, the telephone, the teddy bear, and the therapist and to express this relationship clearly in a complete sentence.

A six-year-old, previously diagnosed as autistic, demonstrated unusual thought processes. In response to "How old are you?" he replied "I have a five." He was able to follow one simple instruction but could not handle two sequential instructions at the same time. For example, he could unerringly point to the larger of two squares and could draw a circle. But when asked to draw a circle inside the big square, he immediately drew a circle outside the big square. Therefore, it seemed reasonable to conclude that this deficit may have accounted for some if not all of the child's strange sentence structure. This is *not* autism!

Affect

The general theory of affect was discussed in Chapter 2. Here, our concern is clinical data that will have some bearing on our final treatment plan. For example, if a child exhibits little anxiety about his misbehavior, traditional individual therapy is probably contraindicated, but if he seems extremely fearful, the initial goal of therapy will be to establish a feeling of trust.

Motor Skills

Traditionally, motor function has been subdivided into gross and fine skills. A child's gross functioning can be compared with the norms provided in standard developmental tables. If a child can hop on one foot or skip at a certain age, for instance, it is useful to make a general assessment of his clumsiness or agility.

Gross motor coordination can be checked by asking the child to walk, run, stand or hop on one foot, skip, and walk heel-to-toe. His fine motor coordination can be checked by listening to his voice (speech is a fine motor function) and by observing his ability to draw, write, and copy standard figures, perform rapid alternating movements, and the like. A brief neurological screening test for use with children is currently being developed by Mutti, Sterling, Spalding & Crawford (1974).

Memory

Problems involving short-term memory are easily missed, yet may account for serious disorders, as illustrated in the case of the boy who could not follow sequential instructions. Silver (1976) points out that it is essential to identify the child who can carry out a number of individual tasks but cannot link them together. This child will inevitably encounter tremendous difficulties with parents and teachers!

Perception and Perceptual-motor Skills

Assigning a grim diagnosis such as schizophrenia or severe retardation to a child suffering a hearing or visual loss is one of the greatest tragedies in the mental health field:

> A ten-year-old, the third of four sons in a lower middle-class family, was unruly and argumentative both in school and at home. He attacked other children for minimal provocation and seemed comfortable in his role as a bully. The school was extremely upset by his behavior and the situation at home was deteriorating. My initial impression was that the case would require intensive and lengthy therapy, preferably with both the identified patient and his family. The teacher suggested that the child's vision be checked since he seemed to have difficulty seeing distant objects. Within a few days after receiving glasses, the child's behavior improved dramatically, both at home and at school.

A rough auditory test should always be carried out in the office in any case where slow mental development is suspected. This can be done by making soft noises behind the child's back. Although tuning forks are preferable, of course, it is possible to produce middle frequency sounds by rubbing the thumb and forefinger together.

FAMILY'S BEHAVIOR DURING CONJOINT SESSIONS

After an initial evaluative session with the child and parents to gather basic information about the chief complaint, developmental history, and general nature of the family-child system, a conjoint family session is the diagnostic move of choice in most cases. There are excellent reasons for conducting a conjoint session. First, the reports of one individual about the behavior of another are notoriously unreliable. Second, the clinician can obtain at least an inkling of the type of interactions that occur between the family and the identified patient at home.

A diagnostic family session, then, is advantageous for several important and obvious reasons: (1) it clarifies the chief complaint, (2) it clarifies the roles and general patterns of behavior in the family and (3) it provides immediate information about the nature of parental interactions and child discipline, general personality patterns, and so forth. Most important, however, the clinician can use the conjoint session to emphasize both verbally and behaviorally, that although he chooses to see one family member individually as the identified patient, the functioning of the total family system is important, even when the identified patient's dysfunction is clearly the primary focus of treatment. This helps to minimize consolidation of the Sickie role that is often the inevitable price the individual pays for becoming a patient. Is the identified patient, in his family's eyes, allowed to come, or is he forced to come? Will the family use individual therapy to consolidate its power against the patient?

Major Roles and Patterns

Family roles and patterns are often blatantly apparent in the waiting room, on the way down the hall to the therapist's office, and so forth. The order in which family members walk down the hall and how quickly and enthusiastically, who gives instructions to whom, and who speaks to and for whom enable us to make useful inferences about the family's rules.

> While a family of seven was being evaluated, the five children raced down the hall to the office. Their mother, a large aggressive woman, walked next to the the therapist, bellowing at the children to stop making so much noise. The father followed meekly. In the office, the mother barked orders at everyone; the children responded with giggling and horse-

play. Occasionally, the father feebly attempted to reinforce his wife's orders. This general pattern—in which the power appeared to be concentrated in the mother's hands, although she could not control her children—was observed throughout the session.

Communication

Communication theory is a major field of its own (Watzlawick, Beavin & Jackson, 1967; Reusch, 1953). Clinically, however, it is easiest and most useful to divide communication into content and process—*what* is said and *how* it is said—and to help the family observe this differentiation. This preliminary step is essential if the family is to acknowledge patterns of communication that are clearly repetitive, regardless of the specific issue involved. Because the family tends to focus on the content of an argument, it will miss the critical point that the process of interaction is the same. In other words, the family may believe that it is dealing with a new argument each time and that it has a large number of problems. The clinician can point out that the family is actually dealing with one or two repetitive processes and therefore with only one or two fundamental issues. I illustrate this point to families as follows: "There are lots of different kinds of dough, but it seems you are using only one cookie cutter" or "It is like there is a coach on the bench who keeps calling the play over and over again." The family that recognizes the repetitiveness of a constant underlying process despite variation in content is well on the way to a good therapeutic result.

A description of a conjoint family session must, of course, summarize the major topics of conversation. For instance, what do family members spend most of their time talking about? Do they endlessly berate the identified patient for his misbehavior? Do they berate the therapist for his inability to provide an instant cure? Do they complain about the school or the neighbors?

Haley [1967] demonstrated that the sequence in which a family speaks provides important information. In some families, the sequence is relatively fixed. For example, the father may speak first, a rebuttal by the mother follows, the child then interrupts her.

A fixed sequence may be observable in terms of affect as well as content. For example, a predictable sequence that includes a declarative statement, an angry rebuttal, a tearful rejoinder, and inappropriate laughter which recur in an endless loop, makes it possible, without regard to the content of the interaction, to obtain a rough assessment of how firmly the family is locked into a pathological process.

How does the family present the chief complaint? Here is one form of data that is literally thrust upon us. Few or no questions are required to determine how the family presents its problem; yet strong inferences can sometimes be made from these data concerning family dynamics.

Is the Chief Compaint Coherent?

No.   Yes

What is the focus?

Focus is outside the   Focus is on the   Focus is on the
Family   identified   entire
                               patient   family

If the chief complaint is coherent, the focus may be on the identified patient, the family as a whole, or elsewhere. Each possibility is important.

If the chief complaint is incoherent, our work is cut out for us. Therapy is out of the question, and we may be doing well if we obtain an adequate evaluation. The family may be experiencing a massive crisis, and a thorough evaluation may be impossible until a later time. Measures such as medication or hospitalization may be indicated. A family secret of major homeostatic significance may be close to the surface. Perhaps the family has recently moved, by way of a power shift, into a conflict configuration (see pp. 234). Individual therapy with any family member can either be essential or increase the amount of scapegoating. If incoherence persists, the clinician may be dealing with a permanently chaotic family. If so, limited treatment goals are most appropriate. Or he may be dealing with a "chaosogenic" family, which moves from agency to agency and deals with multiple agencies simultaneously.

Very different possibilities pertain if the chief complaint is highly coherent. If the focus is outside the family, limited treatment goals may be sufficient. For example, the family may state that "We're O.K. but the court said we had to come, so here we are." In this case, communication with the "other part of the system" is clearly essential.

A coherent chief complaint that focuses on the identified patient is common. Certainly, this may be the most reasonable way for a family to present itself to the clinician. How much of the difficulty is related to processes within the identified patient, regardless of environment? How much is related to interaction between the identified patient and the environment? The family has no idea—and neither will we until we investigate the situation. If the focus on the identified patient seems rigid, even in the face of data that contradict the allegations, we may be dealing with a situation where the family has decided to extrude the child. This possibility must be carefully assessed with respect to its severity and reversibility. A clear focus on the identified patient may carry with it the implicit or explicit request for therapy for that individual. Such therapy can be appropriate and necessary, represent a "psychiatric assault" on the identified patient on behalf of the family, or increase or decrease the amount of scapegoating.

Occasionally, the focus will be on the entire family. In these cases, the family is likely to have been coached by a previous therapist! Thus the clinician should proceed by examining the issues in a straightforward manner.

Of special interest is the transition from the second to the third possibility. This shift from "the problem is Johnny's temper tantrums" to "the problem is Johnny's temper tantrums, but they have got something to do with the way his brother picks on him, as much as I sympathize with his brother" is crucial. The family that can tolerate this shift in focus is probably well on its way to a good therapeutic result.

Patterns of Identification: Alliances and Barriers

Minuchin (1974) has pointed out the clinical riches to be found in an analysis of a family's alliances and barriers. These often become clear immediately during a conjoint family session. Occasionally, a specific identification process contains all the information necessary to develop a formulation. The following examples illustrate this point:

> Sharon, age 15, attempted suicide by ingesting a moderate amount of aspirin and was hospitalized. I soon learned that her father, a career army officer, had recently been wounded in Vietnam and had written in a letter that his wound was "close to the heart." From this, Sharon inferred that the shell fragment would travel to his heart and kill him and that by the time she had received the letter, he was dead. In an effort to rejoin him, she had tried to take her own life. I pointed out to her that if her father had survived the initial trauma long enough to find his way to a hospital and write her a letter, she could be quite confident that he was alive and well; furthermore, a shell fragment would not travel through the lung and damage the heart. On hearing this, Sharon leaped out of bed and exclaimed happily: "OK, I'm ready to go home."

> A mother brought her eight-year-old son to the clinic for an evaluation because of his poor academic performance. He and his older sister reflected his mother's Scandinavian appearance and speech: they were blond, blue-eyed, and sharply enunciated their consonants. The mother's second

husband was an American Indian, and the two younger children had his bronze skin, brown eyes, and black hair. The two older children reflected their mother's weepy, depressed behavior while the two younger ones were cheerful and self-confident like their father.

The seating arrangement a family chooses is often a rich source of information. If the chairs are arranged randomly before the family enters the room, seating can be used as a projective test. In some cases, the seating positions and interactions can be translated almost directly into the boundaries and affiliations that Minuchin (1974) described. Most families are unaware that these simple, obvious behaviors are in fact powerful projective tests. In addition, the data may be less contaminated by the observer's presence than is true for other behaviors. For example, when the clinician asks "Do you like your child?" the parents are likely to be far more guarded than they are when choosing their seating position. If the verbal language says yes but the body language says no, one would want to pursue the matter further.

> A family of seven requested an evaluation of their six-year-old son because of his uncontrollable violence at home. When I entered the room, I noted with interest that the boy was seated in the middle of the family circle. This maneuver was consistent with his role as the "center" of his family. When asked "Do you like Eddie?" the parents replied: "Well, doctor, we *love* Eddie very much, but sometimes it is hard to like him because he . . . he doesn't seem to understand how hard we *try* to love him to like him when he makes it so difficult for us. And after all we've done for him!"

Four Parameters of Family Function

When I initially began ranking individual family members in terms of four specific parameters—level of anxiety, capacity to change, role as symptom carrier, and power—this process seemed useful, primarily as a means of describing a family to another clinician. Over a period of time, however, it evolved into such a useful clinical tool that a large part of Chapter 8 is devoted to it.

Affect

Initially, of course, a family will inevitably be ill at ease in the interview situation. When they feel more comfortable, however, it is possible to answer the following question: Is the affect of individual members and the family in general appropriate and variable? What is the predominant mood in the family? Is there coherence of mood? For example, do family members laugh and cry at about the same time? Are some family members outside the general flow of feelings? Are individual members allowed to deviate significantly from the predominant flow of feelings? Exclusion from the predominant affective tone of any group can be brutal, as the following vignette illustrates:

> An asymptomatic family was enjoying dinner together. When the adults laughed at a sophisticated joke, the six-year-old chimed in. His father turned to him suddenly and said: "You don't even know what we're laughing about, do you?" and the boy's eyes filled with tears.

Problem-solving Style

By what means are clinical data organized into a clinically useful formulation? In Chapter 2, I described the concept of problem-solving style at some length. Here, the topic will be reviewed briefly from a clinical viewpoint, emphasizing the psychosexual level and the crucial distinction between preoperational and operational thought. The following cases illustrate how a family's psychosexual level can be inferred from their behavior in the clinical situation:

Stage I issues. A six-year-old boy made a serious suicide attempt and was subsequently referred to the clinic for psychiatric evaluation and treatment. Both his parents were severely depressed. Interviews with the parents indicated the presence of Stage I issues, and the predominant feeling in the family was one of loss and hopelessness. When the identified patient was seen individually for the first time, he sulked in the hallway and refused to enter the playroom. Finally, however, he agreed to go for a walk with the therapist, who steered him toward a grocery store. They returned to the office with oranges, which they ate in silence. During the months that followed, therapeutic maneuvers dealt with enjoying, sharing, and subsequently giving up this gratification.

Stage II issues. The school referred an eight-year-old boy because of his disruptive behavior. During the initial telephone contact with the family, his mother could not decide on an appropriate time for the interview but finally agreed to set a time for the appointment. It became clear during a session with the parents that the mother wielded the power in the family; she tolerated no deviations from her plans.

In play therapy, the identified patient demonstrated an interest in clay and left the session with traces of clay on his hands. He came to the next session carrying a shoe box that contained a pair of rubber gloves and a work shirt, which he carefully put on before playing with the clay. After 18 months of weekly sessions, a power struggle occurred over the therapist's attempt to set limits on the boy's behavior in the playroom. At this point, the mother insisted that "He hasn't changed the least bit," while the school reported considerable improvement. The family became chaotic and terminated the boy's therapy.

Stage III issues. An eight-year-old boy was brought to the clinic for an evaluation following a suicide attempt. During a series of interviews with the parents, we learned they had severe sexual problems: the husband described his wife as alternately seductive and inaccessible; his wife said he was aggressive, rough, and inconsiderate. Initially the identified patient preferred to play alone rather than with the therapist. Gradually, however, he began to include the therapist in his play, which became increasingly competetive, first between toy soldiers and subsequently with the therapist on the basketball court (French & Steward, 1975).

Changing our focus from affect to cognition, we can argue that a couple's problem-solving style might shed light on their cognitive functioning. Here again, distinguishing between preoperational and operational thought can be extremely useful. Preoperational thought—characterized by magical thinking, egocentrism, an assumption of irreversibility, and a tendency to lump together the many elements of a complex situation—only makes the usual adjustment problems of life more difficult. In contrast, operational thought, which is characterized by the ability to use internal representations of external events in a reversible way, permits rapid and reversible scanning of many options. Furthermore, the capacity to see a complex perceptual field (such as another person) as consisting of a large number of independently variable components makes it possible to deal with interpersonal problems with far more flexibility.

PARENTS' BEHAVIOR

A careful description of the parents' behavior, both individually and together, may begin the required data base. For example, if a patient's mother is massively obese, slovenly, and shabbily dressed, smokes continually, and coughs heavily, her behavior may indicate a tendency to organize her life around immediate gratification of dependency needs. If a patient's father is a meticulously neat man who carefully brushes erasure crumbs off the corner of your desk as he sits down, and obviously feels uncomfortable about the books and papers piled on top of your book case, he may be telling you that issues of control will be important.

The parents' interaction with the identified patient can be described in a similar way. For instance, are they furious with him, and do they intend to throw him out at the first opportunity? Do they like him? Have they been sent to the clinic against their will at the insistence of the court or school system? Are they desperate for help, or are they indifferent?

Although I have never seen a complete, formal examination of a parent's mental status included as in a child-family workup, the parents' affect, attitudes, mannerisms, unusual thought processes, and the like should certainly be noted. Although psychiatrists take great pride in the clinical interview as the core of their diagnostic and therapeutic work, Grinker (1975) stated that "psychiatrists are notoriously poor observers of behavior . . . Clinical psychologists, on the other hand, do observe well, and when reporting test results, describe in great detail the behavior of their subjects [p. 161]." Since the controversy between the "clinical" and "statistical" approaches has been settled on the "statistical" side (Meehl, 1954), a case has been made for the Minnesota Multiphasic Personality Inventory (MMPI). This tool must be used with appropriate clinical sensitivity, however.

Because we do not always have the luxury of unlimited time to spend on an evaluation, an interview with both parents together must compete with the time we spend with the identified patient and with the family in conjoint sessions. Nevertheless, some important information probably cannot be gained in any other way. It has been said that a clinician will not understand a couple until he knows about their sex life. Certainly, a couple's sexual functioning can reveal sensitive aspects of their interaction as no other data can. We can obtain some inkling about how a couple organize their relationship by asking questions such as "Do you like each other? or "Is being together something you get to do or something you *have* to do?" (Obviously, it is rarely appropriate to discuss such marital issues in the presence of children.)

Clinical data about how a couple organize their relationship virtually pour over the clinician in any clinical setting. For example:

> Half way through a session, a father interrupted the flow of his own thoughts by saying to his wife: "Oh, that reminds me. I've got to go to Los Angeles tomorrow. Have you got my shirts ready?" She replied, "Yes, dear."

Although parents are likely to discuss their feelings about the identified patient more openly if he is absent, one might want to bring up this issue in his presence at a later time.

OTHERS IN THE SOCIAL NETWORK

There are several good ways to get into trouble with a case involving a family. One way is to be unaware of a person who exerts a significant amount of influence on the identified patient's life situation. I like to view the identified patient as a ship that is following a course by means of a compass and travels past a series of huge iron deposits. In other words, the identified patient's symptoms make sense only if we understand the complex field through which he is navigating. The iron deposits represent important people in the identified patient's life. If we are unaware of them, we will be unable to understand the patient's behavior. Logically, this point belongs here; operationally, however, I would put it in the chapter about the family tree because it is my custom to ask parents questions such as the following: "Is there anybody else in your family or among your friends whose opinions are extremely important to you, whose friendship you would not want to lose, or whom you would consult about any important decision?" "Is there anyone in your life, in or out of your immediate family, who could make you feel terrible if they thought you had done something silly?" "Do you belong to a church?" "Do you belong to a lodge or a social group of any kind?" When working with an American-Indian family, tribal customs may be of major importance since members of the tribe, although not actually members of the immediate family, certainly may function as such. These individuals, and their significance, should be noted on the family tree.

ADDITIONAL SOURCES OF DATA

Direct clinical observation of children is usually supplemented by reports from teachers and other observers. Special testing on the biological or psychological levels also may be indicated. As we approach this part of the evaluation, the diagnostic possibilities considered should become increasingly specific.

School or day care center. Because teachers and operators of day care centers are often excellent observers of child behavior, they can provide invaluable information about the identified patient's capacity to make friends and relate to teachers and administrators; his participation in extracurricular activities; the attitudes of peers, teachers, and administrators, toward him; and so forth. Therefore, these sources should always be contacted, by phone at least, after the family has granted permission to do so.

Psychological tests. Do not order psychological testing indiscriminately. Any fool can (and often does) use every diagnostic maneuver in the book and then calmly sit back during staff conferences and wait for abnormalities to fall onto the table. This procedure has all the subtlety and aesthetic appeal of shooting a flock of geese with a cannon loaded with buckshot. A more professional approach is to consult with a psychologist about the specific differential diagnostic considerations involved in the case and leave it to his professional discretion to choose the appropriate tools. Chapter 7 describes a formulation that is more valuable than a diagnosis. (Those who wish to pursue the specifics of psychological testing further should consult Anastasi, 1968, and Buros, 1970.)

Physical examinations. Although the physical examination is the special province of the physician or nurse-clinician, some areas of physical function can be tested without having the patient undress or be touched. The problem each clinic faces is to put together an appropriate set of tools that will yield maximum information about pathology with a minimum of effort. The complete workup, carried out without regard for expense or difficulty is, in a way, a trivial problem. But evaluating a large number of high-risk children within a reasonable period and at reasonable cost is a challenge!

A clinician of any discipline can note the following physical characteristics. Does the child look well developed and well nourished? Does he look strange? As Wender points out, many high-risk children fall into "an accurately described pediatric subgroup . . . [called] 'FLK' or funny-looking kid (1971, p. 29)." Autistic children, on the other hand, are classically described as beautiful and graceful. Fish (1971) has described in detail the unstable autonomic, motor, and metabolic functions that characterize schizophrenic children.

Height and weight are sensitive indicators of the child's nutritional and metabolic state. Therefore, if a child with parents whose height and weight are normal demonstrates a normal growth curve and looks well developed and well nourished, he is unlikely to have a metabolic abnormality severe enough to account for a significant portion of a major behavioral disturbance. On the other hand, if the child's height and weight are significantly below normal, a wide variety of emotional and biological problems must be considered.

Although the nuances of neurological functioning are the province of the specialist, a nonneurologist, and even a nonphysician can watch or test for localized deficits, overall clumsiness or agility, hemisphere dominance, and visual and auditory impairments. For instance, a history of lapses of attention or consciousness, with or without convulsions, may suggest epilepsy. A child usually experiences a basic neurological examination as an enjoyable game. A set of neurological tests suitable for screening purposes has been developed by Mutti et al. (1974).

Laboratory data. Specific laboratory studies may be suggested by positive findings obtained during interviews with a family. A family history of diabetes, growth disturbances, and irritability may indicate diabetes. A neurological examination and history may require an electroencephalogram. A family history of allergy may indicate specific testing if the child shows physical manifestations of allergy. A history of pica and findings that suggest a neurological dysfunction may indicate screening for lead poisoning. It is important to prepare the child for the stress of some laboratory tests. A glucose tolerance test, for example, requires repeated blood samples and confines the patient (and usually a parent) to the laboratory for several hours without food. An electroencephalogram may be essential, but it can be terrifying to the unprepared child. The primary clinician can be enormously helpful in preparing the child for the procedure.

Other agencies and therapists. Other agencies and previous therapists should be contacted routinely. This is essential to the entire management plan in the case of a "chaosogenic" family that simultaneously maintains contact with a large number of agencies and therapists, skill-fully playing them off against each other. (I have coined the term chaosogenic for this ability to create chaos within and between agencies.)

This chapter has briefly discussed the actual "laying-on-of-eyes-and ears" in four sections: waiting room behavior, playroom behavior, family behavior in conjoint sessions, and parental behavior. As a friend once said: "People are more interesting than anybody." Interviewing is a great privilege for the clinician and a wonderful art form. Enjoy it.

Chapter 7

CASE FORMULATION AND
TREATMENT PLAN

Having laboriously collected our data, we can now assemble the pieces of the puzzle and seek to formulate a diagnosis with sufficient explanatory power to make sense of the patient's symptoms as coping maneuvers in the context of his life. A formulation is like a three-dimensional map that explains why water flows in the direction that it does; it presents the family's definition of uphill and downhill.

This chapter covers four topics: evaluating the identified patient, evaluating the family, analyzing current symptoms, and planning treatment strategies. These practical considerations are based on the theoretical material contained in Chapter 2. Although some of this material, such as temperamental type, has already appeared many times, the emphasis here is on viewing symptomatic behavior in a biological, developmental, and situational context.

However, before launching into these specific areas, I want to repeat a warning that appeared in Chapter 2. Beware the power of diagnostic labels! Ideally, the diagno-

sis should be a differential diagnosis—that is, a list of possibilities, ranked according to their probability—and the
basis for each consideration should be specified in terms of
observations clearly presented in the evaluation. This gives
the reader the opportunity to reexamine the data and arrive
at an independent judgment concerning the diagnosis. Too
often, diagnosis is an *ex cathedra* judgment, the basis for
which is unclear although the data presented may be extensive. Remember that seeking help from a professional
helper is not a disease. There is such a thing as normality!

I strongly believe that serious diagnoses such as
schizophrenia and autism should be used with the utmost
care, especially when applied to the young. Finally, keep in
mind that a diagnosis applies to the *least* functional aspects
of the individual's life; therefore, it should be part of a
comprehensive formulation that presents a somewhat
more comprehensive picture than is possible with a single
diagnostic term.

Evaluating the Identified Patient

There are a variety of ways of looking at an individual. Each
is a special clinical tool that may be useful in a specific case.
Each provides a uniquely valuable perspective. Here as
elsewhere, I have attempted to outline concisely the essential features of each viewpoint while recognizing that each
merits a book of its own.

Temperamental Type

In the context of the formulation, we must be alert to the
possibility that the identified patient's temperament has
been a major factor in the development of his symptoms.
Therefore, evidence for the presence of specific traits such
as high activity level, high intensity of reaction, low rhyth-

micity, or poor adaptability, which have contributed significantly to the development of the current situation should be discussed. For example:

> Mrs. L described her five-year-old son, Abe, as "unbearable and unmanageable"; his preschool teacher believed that he was "emotionally disturbed." Abe had always been an extremely active child: his mother had felt him bumping and kicking early in the seventh month of gestation. A high activity level had been reported by all observers and was most obvious in the office. In addition, his history clearly indicated a low threshold to stimuli (i.e., he was a "hair-trigger kid") and intense reactions to stimuli (i.e., his emotions tended to be "full scale," no matter whether he was laughing or crying). Mr. and Mrs. L had been separated intermittently for three years. Mrs. L described herself as "worn out and depressed."

None of these factors was in itself unusual or abnormal. But the combination of factors formed a consistent pattern of interaction between mother and child. Abe would approach his mother and demonstrate his typically high level of activity, low threshold, and high intensity of reaction. Mrs. L, fearing another exhausting interaction, would try in any way she could to avoid it. At this point, Abe's anxiety would increase, and like any adaptive organism, he would attempt to correct the problem by redoubling his effort. Finally, Mrs. L would appease him by offering him candy. The result was an obnoxious, negativistic, tantrum-prone brat who tyrannized his exhausted, depressed mother.

GAP and DSM-II Classifications

GAP report No. 62 (Group for the Advancement of Psychiatry, 1966) is a milestone in the field of child psychiatry. It divides childhood behavioral disorders into the following ten categories: (1) healthy responses, (2) reactive disorders, (3) developmental deviations, (4) psychoneurotic disorders, (5) personality disorders, (6) psychotic disorders, (7) psychophysiologic disorders, (8) brain syndromes, (9) mental retardation, and (10) other. The entire manual focuses on the child as an adaptive organism with its own unique and specific strengths and liabilities, which responds to the specific and unique strengths and liabilities of its environment. The manual is essential for everyone working with children and deserves careful reading. The first four categories—normal, healthy response, adjustment reaction, and developmental deviation—are not diagnoses in the traditional medical sense and reflect a useful broadening of our understanding of disease processes.

The category "developmental deviation" is especially valuable for two reasons: first, it permits the clinician to express serious concern about the possible loss of reversibility of a maladaptive behavior pattern without using the more serious and potentially damaging labels of neurosis and personality disorder, which by definition imply a significant compromise of reversibility. Second, this category permits a fine-grained description of the specific area in which the deviation is located. The splatter effect of most psychiatric diagnoses is thus avoided. This diagnosis might be supplemented by an indication of conditions for which the child is at risk. For example, "developmental deviation in the dimensions of social and language function. At risk for personality disorder, schizoid type and possibly schizophrenia." Or "developmental deviation in the dimension of affective function. At risk for development of neurotic disorder, depressive type." The name of the game is to maximize communication to other clinicians while minimizing the damaging potential of labels.

The GAP manual also includes a comprehensive list of symptoms that facilitates specific descriptions of the target symptoms that concern us.

The official classification system of the American Psychiatric Association (Committee on Nomenclature and Statistics) can be found in *DSM-II: Diagnostic and Statistical Manual of Mental Disorders.* This system is often required for hospital charting.

Psychosexual Development

Chapter 2 discussed psychosexual development in terms of a probability estimate. In other words, given a randomly selected adaptational challenge, does the individual consistently assume that the important issues will be those of a specific developmental level? Because this probability estimate may vary as a function of circumstances, we can talk about optimal and predominant levels:

Optimal level of functioning. What is the identified patient's highest level of function? Although we focus on areas of conflict, our patients may function normally in some areas. For example, an adolescent may spend much of his time arguing with his parents about what are essentially earlier developmental issues (e.g., trust or autonomy), but in another situation, he may demonstrate an age-appropriate ability to address the issue of differentiating himself from the nuclear family and forming a mature identity.

Predominant level of functioning. The contrast between optimal and predominant psychosexual levels gives essential information about the child's dynamic properties, including the ease with which regression occurs, the types of stress that are most likely to cause regression, and the developmental levels to which regression is prone to occur. In other words, is it highly probable that the child will approach a problem assuming that the issues of an earlier developmental stage are of primary importance?

Major Identifications and Introjections

In some cases, children have obviously identified with one parent, incorporating both his strengths and weaknesses.

This fact is useful in formulating a diagnosis as well as in therapy for several reasons. First, evidence of introjection with little modification may indicate an extremely low degree of differentiation between parent and child. Second, if much of the child's behavior, healthy as well as pathological, results from the introjection of an adult, therapy may involve a depressive response because it will be necessary for the child to grieve the loss of the introjected parent before new introjects can form. Change in the child, through therapy or in some other way, may be difficult for the parent and present serious implications with regard to the clinician's approach to both parent and child.

Genetic-dynamic Factors: Major Intrapsychic Conflicts and Their Developmental Origins

Here our concern is intrapsychic conflict between drives or impulses on one hand, a repressive system on the other, and the specific developmental, or genetic roots of the conflict.

> Fourteen-year-old Larry was brought to the clinic because of his outbursts of violent behavior. He alternated, often within seconds, between hugging and striking other family members. His mother had held Larry to her, day and night, sleeping or doing housework, until he was 18 months old. At that time, a second child was born and Larry was abruptly left on his own. Because his mother disliked the sight of a child carrying a bottle, Larry had to fend for himself at the family table as best he could and was fed by other members of the family. On the basis of these and other data, we inferred that Larry's outbursts were related to anger that was appropriate to his abandonment at 18 months after mothering that had undercut any opportunity for development of normal individuation. We hypothesized a conflict between his desire to express his rage and his wish to be close to family members.

Twelve-year-old Hank was referred for evaluation because of his poor performance at school. He was an only child; his parents had divorced during his infancy. Because Hank had been ill many times during infancy and childhood, his mother had in effect run an intensive care unit for him continuously for the first five years of his life, checking on his state of health at hourly intervals day and night. Despite his average intelligence, Hank seemed unable to perform the simplest school work satisfactorily. We inferred that issues of trust and separation (Stages I and II) were active enough in this boy's life to have some bearing on his school failure. Specifically, we hypothesized that functioning well in school may have posed a threat to the close tie between mother and child. Subsequent clinical observation confirmed that despite her vigorous efforts to encourage Hank, his mother simultaneously gave him clear and explicit orders to fail. Therefore, we suspected a conflict between his normal drives for maturation and individuation on the one hand and his wish for closeness on the other.

Bill, an adolescent with a good school record, suddenly began to have "memory problems" during examinations, and his grades deteriorated seriously. His developmental history indicated that nothing unusual had occurred during Stages I and II. When Bill was 3½, however, his father developed cancer and killed himself two years later. During therapy, we found evidence to support the hypothesis that there was an association between issues of initiative versus guilt [Stage III] of childhood (which was exacerbated by the father's death) and Bill's subsequent difficulties at school. We hypothesized that school work represented his capacity to take the initiative in situations and that he was trying to reduce what he perceived to be his excessive power.

A talented young artist had chronic problems with his instructors and behaved obnoxiously during his first major exhibit, which he described as a disgusting ordeal. He was the only child of somewhat elderly parents who, since his early childhood, had given him every possible encouragement and opportunity. During therapy, the artist commented: "I guess I felt like they liked me for my *what* rather than for my *who*." We inferred that the issues of Stage IV (industry versus inferiority) were important in his life and that he was confused about the association between his self-esteem and his work.

Economic Factors: Distribution and Availability of Intrapsychic Resources

Because the energy of all organisms is limited and because this energy is distributed between internal conflicts, external coping mechanisms, and conflict-free activities such as play, excessive demands related to internal conflict will render play impossible and external coping mechanisms ineffective. In other words, we can conceptualize a hierarchy of priorities for the use of energy. The first priority is given to internal balance, the second to the balance between organism and environment, and the third to play. The economic description is an estimate of energy the individual distributes among these priorities. In a child's case, the constant demand for enough energy to adapt to the internal and external challenges of ongoing growth make this assessment especially critical. A moderate reduction of the child's capacity to function in diverse areas of life may be a far more significant indicator of serious difficulties than a complete inability to function in one clearly delineated area, if other areas of function remain good. For example:

An adolescent boy came to the clinic at his parents' insistence because of his drinking, marijuana smoking, staying out late with friends, and sexual activity. Initially, the differential diagnosis included normal peer-group behavior. His previous school performance and peer relationships had been excellent. However, a detailed history revealed that his school performance had deteriorated abruptly and drastically during the last semester; that he had stopped participating in athletics, which had previously been important to him; and that his overall mood had changed. The pervasive nature of the disturbance shifted the diagnostic focus from normality and raised a number of biological and psychological possibilities.

In general, the capacity to cope adaptively with a variety of stresses and a variable, comfortable, and content-appropriate affect indicate that the individual's energies are not being soaked up by intrapsychic conflict. The fixed, cheerful affect or the fixed, friendly manner may be traps for the unwary. The emerging literature on depression in children is of particular interest here (see Malmquist, 1971; Cytryn & McKnew, 1972). *Depression may be the most commonly missed psychopathological state in children.* As in adults, depression in children can be reflected in virtually any symptom picture. A high activity level; a withdrawn, passive state; school performance that is not consistent with ability; aggressiveness or boistrousness may reflect depression.

Major Assets and Liabilities

Personhood can be considered on many levels. The general objective of an evaluation is to estimate the fraction of variance from normality that can be attributed to each level. In child psychiatry, more than in any other area of medicine, a careful examination of each level is essential.

In some cases, strong interactions between levels may illuminate the problem even further. In proposing discrete levels to which we assign names, we run the risk of simplistically dividing the system into isolated parts. The boundaries between levels are selectively permeable in ways that are characteristic of the boundary and the organism, and causality moves in both directions across these boundaries. For example, consider the ancient and tiresome functional-organic and nature-nurture distinctions. The structure of the nervous system has much to do with the nature of the environment, and the environment influences the structure of the nervous system.

Operationally, the biological, psychological, family, and social levels can be useful. Although some clinicians lump the family and social levels together, there is a significant difference between the two in the majority of cases. To illustrate the usefulness of separating these four levels of organization, I will present two case histories and then chart the assets, liabilities, target problems, and interventions related to each in a separate table for each child (see Weed, 1973, 1975; Mazur, 1974).

> The school referred eight-year-old Robert to the clinic because of his intermittently violent behavior. His mother had divorced his father when Robert was an infant and had remarried when he was three years old. His three-year-old half-sister was the darling of both parents. According to his mother, Robert had always been a difficult child, and he fit the description of the difficult temperament. Although his stepfather verbally expressed interest in adopting the boy, his behavior indicated ambivalence about doing so. Robert's drawings of the family suggested enormous conflict about the legitimacy of his place in the home and the role his family might find appropriate for him.

Robert's case can be summarized as follows (it is interesting to note that socially he functioned well, e.g., he had good friends and was active in sports): p. 178.

> Seven-year-old Sandra C had been placed in a special class because she suffered from a severe seizure disorder. Mrs. C had suffered from a similar disorder all her life and repeated attempts to control Sandra's seizures were thwarted by her inability to make appointments, administer medication consistently, and so forth. We speculated that Mrs. C found gratification in sharing this terrible experience with Sandra.

Sandra's case is outlined below: Note that the girl had a good relationship with her sister and with teachers and peers. p. 179

This type of tabulation often facilitates discussions about complex cases. Too often, a multidisciplinary staff conference deteriorates into a tug of war if the case presents difficulties on several levels. The operational task is to estimate not only the variance from normality that is attributable to events at each level but the cost of intervention at each level. A rough estimate of the cost/benefit ratio often facilitates treatment planning.

Strong interactions between levels also can be important. For example, a handicapped child born into a family that is prone to play the Game of Rescue (Berne, 1964) would be involved in strong interactions between the biological and family levels.

EVALUATING THE FAMILY

Formulating a diagnosis of the family is an emerging area within child and family psychiatry (Tseng et al., 1976; Ackerman, 1967; Ackerman & Behrens, 1974; Ackerman & Sobel, 1950). In this section, which outlines a general conceptual means of devising this type of formulation, the family will be discussed first as a system and then as an environment.

The Family As a System

To arrive at a formulation about the family as a system, we must first identify the rules that govern the interactions among family members; i.e., the family rules of adaptation. These rules fall into two categories: those pertaining to Type I processes and those pertaining to Type II processes.

RULES OF ADAPTATION RELATED TO TYPE I PROCESSES.   In Chapter 1, Type I processes were defined as relating to a

Level	Assets	Liabilities	Target Problem	Intervention
Biological	Strong; good health	Difficult temperament	None	None. (Some would recommend drug therapy for his hyperactivity)
Psychological	Good intelligence	Strong tendency to negativistic behavior: Stage I anxieties? Stage II difficulties related to father's departure when Robert was 3?	Negativistic behavior	Individual therapy if intrapsychic conflict seem predominant and if scapegoating can be avoided.
Family	Good relationship with mother and half-sister.	Conflict about "legitimacy"; stepfather has not adopted him legally or emotionally	Lack of clarity concerning family membership	Family counseling directed specifically to this issue; conjoint family therapy if family is interested and if counseling is ineffective
Social and institutional	Capable of long-term friendships; involved in sports	Prone to power struggles with adults in position of authority	Power struggles with teacher	Discuss Robert's situation with teacher and principal, avoiding the implication that they are at fault, and look for ways to catalyze improvement

Psychosexual Level	Assets	Liabilities	Target Problem	Intervention
Biological	Good overall health; easy temperament, good mood and adaptability	Seizure disorder.	Seizures	Medication
Psychological	Average intelligence, good self-esteem	Conflict about loyalty to mother: sick child vs. desire for personal growth	Mother's covert agenda of sharing experience with Sandra	Individual therapy, possibly followed by group therapy
Family	Older sibling; mother's agenda-free areas of concern for Sandra	Mother's covert agenda that Sandra share her experience	Mother's covert agenda	Involve mother in group of parents with similar problems, or in individual counseling or therapy concerning her covert agenda; conjoing family therapy to explore intra-familial value of Sandra's seizures
Social and institutional	Good relationships with teachers and a few peers. Likeable.	Social stigma related to frequent seizures, which required that she wear a helmet.	Social stigma of seizures	Talk to Sandra's school class; assist the school in any feasible way.

system with stable reference points. The rules governing Type I processes therefore involve the maintenance of the organism's critical parameters near these reference points, which are provided by the family mythology. Because Type I processes do not require changes in the family mythology, changes in family roles are unnecessary. Thus these processes are relevant to counseling rather than to therapy. Many families, especially those with a psychotic member, are apparently capable of Type I processes alone.

Amount of deviation permitted. How far can an individual deviate from the behavior required by a role before the family will seek to correct this deviation? The following case history illustrates that even minute deviations propel some families into an uproar:

> Mrs. F, in a state of great agitation, brought "uncooperative" 16-year-old Judy to the clinic. There was no history of psychiatric disorder in the family, and Judy was a good student, had friends, and participated actively in extracurricular activities. She was likable, attractive, neatly dressed, and well groomed and viewed her mother's concern about her behavior as ridiculous. The precipitating event was an argument that had occurred when Judy wanted to drink tea. Mrs. F insisted that she drink milk, and Judy angrily left the house, saying "I'm going to my friend's house" and stayed there two hours longer than usual. Mrs. F interpreted Judy's behavior as a sign of incorrigibility and became extremely anxious. Clearly, this family permitted a minimal amount of deviation. Thus Judy precipitated a crisis with an infraction that would seem trivial to the casual observer.

Probability that deviations will be corrected. Children respond to their parents' behavioral rather than verbal messages. Thus parents who complain that their children "don't mind" them are often the ones who follow through inconsistently on promises and threats. This lack of consistency may force the child to create chaos so that he can clarify the rules on a particular day. The child's situation is similar to that of an executive who must make decisions and predictions based on limited data. Information is extracted best from a system that is in motion, if not in crisis. Inconsistencies require repeated samplings to obtain a probability estimate in which one can have reasonable confidence. Therefore, the confused child who perceives that there is a significant discrepancy between his parents' verbal and behavioral statements and has learned to mistrust verbal information must generate turbulence to determine the family structure. The child's confusion will be exacerbated if he has a learning or memory disorder.

Consequences of correcting deviations. My strong clinical hunch is that families which are most prone to be inconsistent about correcting behavioral deviations are also most prone to use vigorous or violent corrective measures. Families often oscillate along this dimension: i.e., the initial threat of vigorous measures is subsequently modified when the parents' rage is replaced by guilt. For example:

> A middle-aged father angrily berated his preadolescent son, Herb, for failing to help with household chores. As we examined the disciplinary process, it became clear that the father initially asked Herb to participate, then demanded that he participate, then threatened what would happen if he did not participate, and finally helped Herb perform the task and in such a way that the father did most of the work. Therefore, the father's behavioral message was "Wait 'til I'm ready to help you."

In other words, there are two extremes of correcting deviations from role-appropriate behavior. At one extreme is a random, vigorous, or violent correction of both minute and large deviations; at the other extreme is consistent use of moderate means to correct deviations.

RULES OF ADAPTATION RELATED TO TYPE II PROCESSES.   Type II processes involve shifts in the reference system with respect to which a system is functioning. In families, the reference system consists of a set of roles, which are established by the family mythology (Ferreira, 1963). The following issues are relevant to this discussion: role clarity, rules for changing the family mythology, and the consequences of changes in the family roles or mythology.

Role clarity. In any system, a lack of clear reference points guarantees chaos. Therefore, it follows that a lack of role clarity guarantees chaos in any family. As a child matures, his role must be defined constantly. The Oedipal complex can be conceptualized as a problem of role clarity. Families are divided along lines of generation and sex, and these boundaries must not become confused. The child who encounters difficulty with the family triangle may be puzzled by a request that he fulfill functions which are inappropriate for his age.

Rules for changing the family mythology. Although useful, valid generalizations are hard to come by, the following may be a good one: Any organism—whether an individual, a family, or a social system—will carefully protect its reference system and will have stringent rules for changing that reference system. At the biological level, mutations in the DNA occur slowly. At the psychological level, self-images and introjects change slowly. At the family level, the core belief structure changes slowly. And at the socioinstitutional level, changes in constitutions occur only occasionally.

An organism's inability to change its reference structure will ultimately result in death. If the structure is not adequately protected from outside influences, chaos will result. For instance, the individual who makes frequent, chameleon-like changes in his personality seems to lack an essential self.

The rules governing changes in the reference structure may be deeply buried, and careful observation and testing of hypothesis over a long period may be necessary to ferret them out. One critical rule concerns the number of Type I maneuvers a family must undergo before it will consider a Type II maneuver. In other words, how close must the family come to a breakdown of homeostasis before resorting to an alternative process? For example, a family may make a change only after a massive crisis. That is, all Type I maneuvers must be exhausted before it will consider a Type II maneuver. A more adaptive family, on the other hand, might make a Type II maneuver before it is threatened with complete breakdown.

Another rule may require the approval of a person in power before a structural change is possible. For this reason, is it essential to search the family tree carefully at the outset for individuals who wield the most power in a family. The clinician who fails to do so may be caught flatfooted in the middle of treatment as the person in power announces behaviorally: "I do not approve of the changes which are occurring in the family structure. Cease and desist!" The family must then grieve the loss of the powerful person's influence (i.e., increase the degree of differentiation within the family—an arduous task) or, bowing to his influence, terminate treatment in some way. This process will be discussed extensively in Chapter 8.

How does one determine what the rules are for changing the family mythology? One clever way is to ask. If asked too soon, such a question could be nonproductive and potentially damaging. However, after careful observation —and if the working alliance with the family is adequate and one is reasonably confident in his working hypothesis —it may be appropriate to share one's working hypothesis with the family, carefully observing its responses at all levels.

Consequences of changes in roles and family mythology. Some families, particularly poorly differentiated ones, behave (perhaps realistically) as though a major change in the role of a family member will be disastrous for part or all of the family. Numerous examples of drastic and sometimes destructive changes that occur after one family member changes attest to the validity of this concern.

On the social level, change in the family core mythology can affect the family's relationship to the entire extended social network and therefore be prohibitively expensive. In general, a small Type II change—a small shift in the system's mythology—requires a tremendous amount of Type-I work as the entire system adjusts to the new reference structure. For instance, changing a few sentences of the Constitution sometimes necessitates decades of readjustment throughout society. We are quick to anger when an individual or family demonstrate clinical "resistance." Perhaps this resistance reflects the organism's wisdom concerning the immense labor involved in change. Given the choice between the myth that the identified patient "got sick all by himself" and a lifetime of readjusting to a new reality, how many of us would choose the latter without some resistance?

Again, one can gain some understanding of the family's belief structure concerning the consequences of a change in the core mythology by asking, at a clinically appropriate point: "How do you imagine the family would respond if Billy changed?" During therapy, it is essential to observe a family closely for evidence of a realignment of roles and alliances. Often, the family will present this material fleetingly toward the end of a session. The process is fairly predictable. First, the family complains in a variety of ways to the clinician that the child's symptoms are becoming worse. This reflects the failure of Type I (homeostatic) processes and heralds the onset of a crisis. Finally, often toward the end of a session and cushioned with joking or another form of uproar, the family presents evidence of a fundamentally new configuration. The clinician should, at this point, watch carefully for evidence of a new process, a new set of alliances, or a shift in roles. When any of these

occur, he should immediately try to find out how it occurred, and, most important, how the family members feel
about the new configuration. If everyone feels better, the
configuration may be stable and represent improvement. If
some family members feel better and others feel worse—
the clinician must try to work with those whose position is
threatened.

A general principle is emerging here. If the family
presents Type I processes, watch for information. If new
behavior indicates a Type II process, stop and dig for more
information, particularly about affect.

Generally speaking, the clinician alone will detect the
enormous importance of an apparently trivial event. The
woman who, for the first time in her life, seasons the soup
differently than her mother did deserves appropriate recognition and support for what may have been a crucial and
heroic undertaking. The intensity of the interaction is irrelevant; it is the *form* of the interaction that is important.

ROLES AND FAMILY MYTHOLOGY.   So far, I have outlined
six general processes whereby the family functions as a
system. Here, our concern is the specific roles that are
assigned to family members. Some common roles are clear:
e.g., the scapegoat and its opposite, the rescuer who is
above reproach. Other roles, such as the "sparkplug" (the
unobtrusive but effective child who triggers chaos at crucial
moments) tend to be more subtle. The schedule of selective reinforcement by which roles are maintained may involve a discrepancy between verbal and nonverbal
communications or statements that destroy the legitimacy
of contrary data. For example, if a family is maintaining a
youngster in the role of "Lazy Kid," an interaction between
parent and therapist might sound like this: "Mrs. Jones,
you've complained that Eddy is lazy—that's why you've
brought him here. His brother just now told all of us that
he mowed the lawn this weekend." "Well, yes, he did—but

only because he knew he couldn't go swimming unless. . . ." In other words, Mrs. Jones has just disavowed, or rendered irrelevant the fact that Eddy actually mowed the lawn. The evolution of a role ("He's been lazy since he was born. The doctor had to slap his ass four times to get him to cry") and family affect around changes in Eddie's behavior ("Wow, he's changed," versus "Yes, but. . . .") help us to understand how firmly embedded roles can be in the family structure.

Content of roles. The identified patient may be labeled scapegoat and a sibling may be labeled peacemaker; one parent may be labeled the representative of law and order while the other is "not involved."

> In a family of nine, there were four boys and three girls. The girls functioned well but all the boys had been involved in a variety of serious difficulties. Two had been institutionalized on a long-term basis. The identified patient was the youngest boy. The parents agreed that "the girls have more sense and seem to do better, while the boys are all too headstrong to raise right."

Although the flow of causality in this family was no doubt complex, as always it was clear that by the time we saw the family, the roles for male and female children were clear and firmly set. The family tree usually provides essential information about the content of roles.

Relationship of roles to current crisis: adaptive and maladaptive roles.

In the case of a transient stress reaction that is clearly caused by external stress, we would ordinarily expect to find an adaptive relationship between roles and the presenting crisis. On the other hand, we would usually expect to uncover a maladaptive relationship between the family mythology and the presenting problem if the symptoms have evolved gradually and are syntonic to the family. For example, in the family just described, the boys consistently ran amuck and the girls consistently functioned well. There is probably some relationship between the family role structure and the identified patient's presenting symptoms. Symptoms of anxiety and depression in the identified patient and behaviors such as running away could be healthy responses if the growing child seeks to rebel against family pressures to fill a role that is expensive and maladaptive for him.

COMMUNICATION.   The questions to answer concerning a family's style of communication involve the following issues: Is the communication clear? Is it appropriate to the current crisis? The importance of clear communication has been discussed extensively by Reusch (1953), Watzlawik and his colleagues (1967), and Mishler and Wexler (1966). Can family members communicate directly and clearly about important issues? Can they exchange *new* information? Can they exchange information—particularly new information—about their essential belief structures? Can they communicate their feelings?

The conceptual model presented throughout this book is that the symptoms which are of primary concern to mental health professionals—namely, those which are syntonic to the family—tend to persist unless there is at least a minimal restructuring of the family mythology with a resultant change in roles. In clinical terms, the question is: "Can the family discuss the emotionally loaded material reflected in the identified patient's symptomatic behavior? If a family is unable to deal with an emotionally loaded topic, it can avoid doing so in a variety of ways, such as plunging into uproar; using humor, the disruptive behavior of the youngster who serves as the sparkplug, or prolonged silences; or by attacking the therapist, the identified patient, and so on. Certainly, the clinician should explore this sensitive material as respectfully and cautiously with a family as he would with an individual patient.

PROBLEM-SOLVING STYLE.   When evaluating a family's problem-solving style, the following questions are relevant: Does the family confront problems directly? Does it immediately resort to scapegoating? Is it able to engage a problem directly? Can it consider alternate routes when seeking the solution to a problem? Does it commonly seek advice from friends and the extended family? If so, is this a resource or a hazard? Does the family become paralyzed by ambivalence to a degree that makes problem-solving difficult? Can it focus on one problem without becoming involved in a mass of intense but nonspecific communication? If the family becomes extremely angry, can it settle down and try again? If so, does it learn from the first effort?

Usually, a family's problem-solving style consists of one or two simple maneuvers, such as becoming angry with the scapegoat or asking the clinician what he intends to do about "this mess." It may be clinically useful to point out to a family how it becomes embroiled in useless problem-solving efforts. Videotape is one excellent method of doing this because it permits an instant rerun of a critical sequence.

A couple who described their children as brats spent the first 20 minutes of a videotaping session insisting that the children focus their attention on "all the problems we have been having." Throughout this battle, the children gleefully engaged in horseplay. Abruptly the mother said: "OK! we will get you ice cream on the way home! And what's more you can just *have it all* your way!" She then sat pouting; her husband was silent. The entire scene was instantly transformed. The children sat down and gave the parents their full attention and a discussion about family issues ensued. By the end of the session, the family had forgotten the sequence of maneuvers that had led to the meaningful discussion. The parents, pleased that they had successfully produced a "laundry list" for the therapist's examination, were irritated when the therapist chose to focus on the family's problem-solving style. With videotape, however, it was possible to show them the radical transformation that had taken place when the mother promised the children ice cream and power. The parents were then able to recognize that this was how they usually interacted with their children.

Mrs. R described six-year-old Herbie as "just a terror at home and at preschool both." The overall pattern of behavior was as follows: Herbie would explore the office, which soon led to what Mrs. R viewed as mischief. She would angrily order him to stop, but he would persist. She would then swat Herbie, who would have a tantrum.

Clearly, this mother-child system had a limited number of intermediate options and relied on a rigid and simple problem-solving method that escalated immediately into a physical altercation. After looking at a videotape of this pattern, Mrs. R realized that Herbie had long ago learned to ignore verbal threats but that he would usually respond if she touched his shoulder or took his hand while firmly suggesting that he change his behavior. In other words, a combination of discipline and affection was most effective.

The Family As an Environment

CAPACITY TO ENSURE PHYSICAL SURVIVAL.   Do the children receive adequate nutrition and health care? Is there a danger of severe physical abuse? Can the family afford to live in safe and appropriate surroundings? Are the children at high risk for severe neglect or abuse? If so, can the parents accept appropriate advice, intervention, and assistance?

CAPACITY TO VALIDATE THE CHILD'S REALITY TESTING AND AFFECT.   Children are not small adults mentally any more than they are physically; they must continually construct and reconstruct their internal representation of reality. Here again, Piaget's concept of preoperational thought (Flavell, 1963) is enormously rich from the clinical viewpoint. If the logic of a preschool child is more qualitative than quantitative and is characterized by egocentrism, magical causality, and the assumption that all events are irreversible, then the four-year-old's incessant questions serve a critical function as the child seeks to construct cognitive tools with which to make sense of the world.

The Piagetian and psychoanalytic psychologies are beautifully complementary and synergistic. For example, the enormous cognitive challenge of the Oedipal complex, namely "Why don't I get to be as close as I would like to the person who is most precious to me?" must be handled with preoperational logic!

Teasing a preschool child can be incredibly brutal. Unfortunately, many adults seem to enjoy boggling the minds of young children. The combination of magical thinking, strangely unreliable and inconsistent adult behavior, and a major overhaul of all cognitive structures may represent the challenge of a lifetime. Teasing a child of this age can be compared to asking a patient afflicted with vertigo "Which way is up?" and then roaring with laughter because he is unable to answer.

Child abuse is not limited to physical injury. Families that conspire to "protect" children from harsh realities often create an impossible conflict. The child perceives one reality, but adults describe a different one. Faced with this dilemma, the child may be forced to disavow his own sense of reality to gain his family's nurture. Examples of this phenomenon are ubiquitous: The weeping mother who says "I feel fine; there's nothing to worry about"; the arguing couple who insist "We're just talking, you kids go to bed"; and the like.

Although the development of affect may forever defy an analysis as rigorous as the one Piaget carried out in the cognitive realm, the same general principles of development probably apply. Namely, the organism actively creates its internal representation of reality through the interaction of intrinsic biological factors and external reality. If we define affect as a set of signals that advises the organism about the survival value of a course of action, then the organism must learn to associate appropriate affects with specific situations. In other words, the child must be able to assess, automatically and accurately, the survival value of different courses of action in a wide range of circumstances.

> After many months of individual therapy for depression, a young man began to describe his family's rules. As inferred from these sessions, the process that developed in his family of origin was as follows: Family members were obligated to care for each other and, through alcoholism and other forms of dysfunction, take turns in the Sickie and Rescuer roles. Because affect was tightly linked to the family process, good feelings were permitted only in the context of the Sickie-Wellie relationship. If a family member had good feelings in another context, he was accused of not caring for the family. If a Sickie began to feel better, he was immediately rejected, felt bad, became a Sickie again, and was reinstated as a good family member. In other words, good feelings were not only restricted to but required in the context of the Wellie-Sickie relationship. Bad feelings were permitted only in, and were absolutely required in the context of separation from and longing for the family.

This system is a common one, particularly in families where the Game of Alcoholism is part of the family process (Berne, 1964). Its essential properties in this patient's life were summarized by the patient's feeling that "It's as though it was the baby's *duty* to cry so that the mother would know she was a good mother." The patient's affect was validated if he affirmed the family myth, and his family tried to undercut his attempts to grow away from this system. In the sense that affect consists of a set of signals which informs us about the survival value of a particular course of action, it is apparent that the meaning of good and bad feelings had been transposed in this family. Therefore, it is no surprise that the patient was profoundly confused about his own feelings and that his interpersonal relationships had a distant quality.

EXISTENCE OF COVERT AGENDAS.   The theoretical assumption that a child's symptomatic behavior may be a direct reflection of deeply hidden parental wishes was discussed in Chapter 1. Johnson (1949) and Szurek (1942), based on studies of juvenile delinquents, wrote classic papers in this area.

The following examples illustrate how parents can actively, albeit covertly, encourage their children to carry out their own forbidden wishes.

> A family sought an evaluation of two sons who were extremely destructive at home. Although the parents claimed to be distressed by the boys' behavior, the father proudly referred to the boys as "my two little tigers."

> An adolescent was brought in for an evaluation of his poor school performance. After berating her son for his poor attitude toward the school, the mother talked at length and with strong feelings about the inadequacies of the school system. She ended by saying "The school is so bad, I just as soon he'd stay home and not go to school at all."

> A four-year-old was brought in because of his "hyperactivity." We soon learned, however, that although he reacted strongly to stimuli when with his parents, he behaved normally under other circumstances. When we contacted the day care center, the director stated: "Now, here is an interesting thing. When the mother brought the child in, she said 'We need a witness [to prove that the boy is bad and incorrigible].' " The parents were incensed by our diagnosis that their son was normal and sought another evaluation elsewhere. We had failed in our objective, which was to acknowledge the family's pain and simultaneously help them to accept the fact that the entire family was involved in the identified patient's problem. If the parents need the child's

misbehavior to express their own inner distress, then the statement, "Your child is normal," may be interpreted to mean "Your feelings are not important, and I do not care about your distress." And if the parents refuse to recognize that the family interaction is part of the problem, the evaluation may well reach an impasse.

Mrs. J sought an evaluation of ten-year-old Charles because he functioned poorly in school and was depressed. It was my impression that Mrs. J and her son were poorly differentiated and that this facilitated her use of projection. Thus applying the label of patient to Charles would enhance this process. Although Charles was indeed symptomatic, treating him individually might confirm the family myth of "sick child." Yet the Js had terminated therapy at two other clinics when it was suggested that the entire family was involved in Charles's problems. Therefore, we saw family members in different combinations for a total of four sessions in the hope that they would eventually accept family therapy. However, our attempts were unsuccessful because we could not establish an adequate working relationship with Mr. J. We then suggested that because Mrs. J and Charles shared a similar type of depression and were extremely close and important to each other, it was essential for Mrs. J to work actively with a therapist, regardless of Charles's need for therapy. She seemed to accept this recommendation but left therapy a few weeks later.

It is not uncommon to discover that the parents of a disturbed child support his symptomatic behavior in a covert way. However, I cannot emphasize strongly enough that a possible causal relationship between family dynamics and the identified patient's symptoms must be handled with extreme care. The statement "the family made him sick" or "the family keeps him sick" is not justified by general system theory; it is basically a demonology model of illness. The relationship between the identified patient's symptoms and family homeostasis must be carefully examined in each case and, if it exists, must be interpreted sensitively to the family.

CAPACITY FOR INTIMACY.   Does anyone have a good definition of intimacy? Whatever intimacy may be, it involves highly coherent communication between two or more people about issues relating closely to the core belief structure of at least one of them. The term highly coherent means that all components of the communication—verbal, intraverbal, and nonverbal—deliver the same message, just as a good piece of art coordinates disparate elements so that the whole is greater than the sum of its parts.

The coherence of a family's communication can be determined by observing whether the different channels of communication mesh. Coherent communication that includes joyful affect takes place between people who *like* each other.

A second element of the capacity for intimacy, the ability to communicate directly about one's core belief structure, can be determined more directly. Often, communication about internal realities has a quality that can be described as clear, calm, and moderately intense. This kind of communication can occur only in an environment of trust and is therefore preceded by a certain amount of waiting and testing. In this sense, intimacy should not be confused with physical proximity.

CAPACITY TO FACILITATE DIFFERENTIATION.   As outlined in Chapter 2, degree of differentiation can be divided into five levels.

Level 1. Families that function at Level 1 are easily identified and their clinical patterns are fairly predictable. In the majority of these families, at least one member is psychotic or suffering from some other severe dysfunction. These families play hard versions of life games. At the lower end of the scale lies symbiotic psychosis; at the upper end lies *folie a deux* patterns and other evidence of shared delusional systems. The concept of "loose ego boundaries"—a term that has been used extensively in connection with schizophrenic patients—applies to this group.

> Mr. V and his girlfriend brought Mrs. V to the emergency room, demanding hospitalization on the grounds that she had "gone crazy again." Mrs. V said, "Well, doctor, at least one good thing has come out of all this. I found out how to have an orgasm." When the clinician asked her to clarify her statement, Mrs. V said: "Why, I know that she [the girl-friend] has orgasms, so I just pretend that I am her, and it works! It's the first time in my life I ever experienced an orgasm." The clinician acknowledged the value of this dis-covery if she was interested in experiencing orgasms. To this, Mrs. V responded with surprise: "Well, that is an aw-fully stupid comment." She then answered his obvious "Why?" with: "Well because then *she* gets the benefit while *I* do all the work."

Level 2. Members of families at Level 2 usually struggle actively to maintain a reasonable degree of autonomy from the nuclear family by active rebellion or hostility or are overly dependent on the nuclear family. They often live near the family, and communication among family mem-bers occupies a large portion of their time and energy. Here, as in Level 1, individuals are often involved in hard versions of life games such as alcoholism. *It is when dealing with Level 2 families that the clinician is prone to overestimate the degree of differentiation. The result is months or perhaps years of work with no discernible results. Generally speaking, these families seem far more differentiated and functional than they actually are.* Although a number of family members function well and are reasonably well differentiated from the nuclear family, one member is highly symptomatic and his symptoms are tightly enmeshed in core family issues. Often, the family will confront the clinician with a unified demand to "straighten out" the identified patient and leave other fam-ily issues alone. Psychoses may be found at the lower end of the range. A higher degree of differentiation may be represented by individuation-separation difficulties such as alcoholism, elective mutism, and school phobia.

Somewhere between the upper part of Level 2 and the lower part of Level 3 there is a crucial water-shed. Families at the lower end of Level 2 will not make structural shifts. Families at the upper end of Level 2 can make significant structural shifts, although usually not without turbulence. Families at the upper end of Level 3 will usually make structural changes without excessive turbulence.

As stressed in Chapter 2, a clinical assessment of families at Level 2 requires great care. The family tree is very useful here. Are there members of the social network whose opinions are crucial to the family? If so, what are the consequences of deviating from family norms. Not uncommonly, one spouse has rejected his own family of origin and fled to the other spouse's family for refuge. This behavior gives all the more weight to the rescuing family's core mythology because there is a lack of alternative role models for family members to follow. Because the component of family interaction that is most relevant to evaluation and therapy is usually the *least* differentiated part of the entire family network, it is not at all uncommon to find, in a family that seems normal in most ways, one area which is in this range of differentiation and where the problem-solving maneuvers are clearly carried out with preoperational logic. At this point, the clinician must carefully inquire in appropriate language whether the family is capable of making the kind of Type II changes necessary to effect a significant restructuring. If it is able to do so, therapy can proceed in that direction, and a new configuration may appear which allows *all* family members to live happier, more adaptive lives. On the other hand, the family may decide that the price of change is too great. In this case, an appropriate goal of therapy would be to help the family outline its limitations and make the best Type I adjustments possible.

Although this kind of assistance is usually viewed as second-class therapy, I strongly believe that we are unfair both to ourselves and to our patients if we insist that everyone who walks through our doors must stay until a sizable Type II change occurs. Some individuals or families can live more comfortably with symptoms that were formerly extremely disturbing if they have an opportunity to assess the alternatives in Type II terms. These families tend to make us angry because they cannot make the Type II changes our therapeutic bias has led us to prefer. We are sometimes amazed to find such a low level of differentiation hidden beneath the layers of normality.

Again, overestimating the degree of differentiation of families at Level 2 is easy to do and leads to chaos. For example:

> Mr. and Mrs. K brought their 12-year-old son, Eddie, to the clinic after he had been caught shoplifting several times. This upper-middle-class, respectable, likable, hard-working, sincere, concerned couple worked hard at the family business and had always tried to maintain a close and loving family. Both parents were proud of what they had achieved despite difficulties in their own families of origin. Mr. K's parents had divorced when he was quite young ("I think he [my father] had a drinking problem") and his mother had remarried when he was ten. His stepfather was "a very good guy" but began to gamble compulsively on an intermittent basis—a pattern that continued until his death a few years earlier. Mr. K's mother was a conscientious woman who attended church "at least twice per week." Mrs. K's mother had died of cancer when Mrs. K was a small child, and Mrs. K had been raised by an elderly, childless aunt and uncle. Initially, the Ks presented us with "We want the very best for Eddie," which they apparently envisioned as residential treatment. They agreed to a combination of individual and family therapy.

The family sessions began with a coherent chief complaint that Eddie was the primary problem. As treatment progressed, the therapist became increasingly angry and frustrated because the family did not perceive that the entire family process was involved to some degree in Eddie's problems. Although some changes for the better did occur, Mr. and Mrs. K continued to insist that Eddie was arbitrarily and willfully mischievous and incorrigible. Session after session, they berated Eddie for his misbehavior and the therapist for his inability to "straighten the boy out." During the twenty-second session, Mrs. K spontaneously described a dream in which Eddie said to her: "I will do anything I can just to make you angry at me." Gradually, the therapist realized that there was a relationship between Eddie's problems and the Game of Rescue, which had been practiced in both parents' families of origin. During the fortieth session, the Ks agreed that there might be come relationship between Eddie's problems and the family structure but that they could not pay the price of the changes required to create a more appropriate environment for him. Shortly after, Eddie was sent to live with relatives in a distant state.

This type of case carries enormous potential for conflict among staff. It is easy for staff members to become embroiled in the family arguments, overidentify with family members, and enact a conflict that is similar to the one occurring in the family itself. Another important point to consider is the enormous stress that a student therapist experiences when the case does not go well—especially if, during the initial case conference, the family was described as well motivated, bright, verbal, and suitable for therapy. Finally, it is difficult to avoid self-recrimination, confusion, and anger toward a family which clearly indicates that it prefers to restrict its efforts to Type I processes rather than undergo the kind of Type II process which would be required for the type of change it initially believed it wanted.

Level 3. A family that functions at Level 3 ordinarily can tolerate the vicissitudes of therapy. For example, a shift of focus from the identified patient's symptoms to the parents' marital problems can occur without having the parents angrily terminate therapy. Although areas of poorly differentiated function can be found, which creates the usual challenges for the therapist, the family will be able to rely on its strengths during the typical crises of therapy. The family will experiment during sessions with different configurations; family members will take their turns on the hot seat without an undue amount of discomfort.

> A couple sought counseling for their 11-year-old son for "lying and stealing." An asymptomatic 14-year-old daughter joined the others in family therapy. Initially, the parents and the daughter attacked the identified patient, but near the end of the second session, the two children jokingly called attention to the fact that their mother was unhappy because the father consistently came home late for dinner. The family then turned its attention quickly to "more important" matters for the remainder of the session. At the third session, the children and the father began teasing the mother for spending money foolishly. The configuration had shifted: the mother was now the identified patient. In subsequent sessions, many configurations occurred, and everyone took at least one turn on the hot seat. The boy's symptomatic behavior stopped.

Levels 4 and 5. Therapy with families at Levels 4 and 5 should proceed relatively smoothly. These families contain members who balance Type I and Type II processes within themselves and thereby avoid complicated role-structures, hidden agendas, and balance bargains. All family members may improve if one member improves.

The term differentiation, as used here, covers a variety of concepts: the capacity to make Type II changes that involve the core reference structure, the capacity to grieve, the capacity to change roles, and the capacity to move away from the family of origin's core belief structure. Therefore, it should not be confused with diagnosis, socioeconomic status, specific presenting picture, or verbal ability. Even a professorship in child psychiatry does not rule out the possibility of a poorly differentiated family of origin!

EXISTENCE OF MAJOR ALLIANCES AND BARRIERS.   In Chapter 4 I alluded to the importance of strong alliances and strong barriers in a family (Minuchin, 1974). These barriers and alliances are usually easy to find. A good way is to ask whether any family members avoid or refuse to speak to each other, always view things the same way, and so on. Again, the chronicity of patterns gives essential information about the system's rigidity.

Family rigidity, a structural issue, does not depend on the specific areas of agreement or discord within the family. It may indicate the family's need to maintain the status quo. The issue of what specific symptoms will be selected if a family member becomes symptomatic (an issue of context) is another matter, however. The number of strong alliances and barriers may provide us with a measure of the family's rigidity, and its choice of symptoms may relate to the specific content of family patterns. A person who angrily disavows his family of origin (strong barrier) is likely to carry into the next family those same patterns or their exact inverse, creating fixed points around which the family dynamics will arrange themselves. The statement "I was so miserable as a child, I am determined that, above all, my children will be happy and have what I didn't have" might arise from a strong barrier and place tyranny in the hands of children. A strong alliance, e.g., "I just adore my mother," raises the possibility of a person in power who establishes family reinforcement schedules. What does the adored mother say about the identified patient and his problems?

ANALYSIS OF CURRENT SYMPTOMS

If a workup is adequate, the relationship of symptoms to the overall family picture and to the identified patient's life should fall from the evaluation like ripe peaches from a tree. Although parents often claim that a child "acts like that for no reason at all," a thorough evaluation should demonstrate that his symptoms represent a reasonable solution to the challenge of maintaining homeostasis in a specific environment. The child perceives this challenge, based on his own unique biological constitution and developmental history. If it does not demonstrate this, either our data or our formulation is inadequate or we are confronted with a new phenomenon.

The categories used in this section—biological disorders, adaptive responses, and maladaptive responses—are not mutually exclusive. For instance, a child may be blind (biological disorder), and exhibit both adaptive and maladaptive responses to life stress.

Symptoms Related to Biological Disorder

This category includes organic brain syndromes, perceptual deficits, congenital malformations, mental retardation related to biological problems, and the like. If only part of a child's difficulty is caused by a biological disorder, the clinician's job is to estimate the extent to which the biological disorder accounts for the difficulty.

Symptoms As Adaptive Responses

The possibility that symptoms are actually adaptive responses should always be considered. Do not assume that the symptom carrier or family is sick. The following criteria are useful to determine whether a patient's symptoms represent an adaptive response: (1) are the symptoms directly related to a perceived stress? (2) do they appear to be reversible; i.e., can they be expected to disappear in a nonstressful environment? (3) and most difficult to determine, do the symptoms represent a new and appropriate behavior that will increase the individual's ability to function in the future? The symptom carrier may be struggling to differentiate himself from the family and be asking for help more vigorously than other family members.

Bowen (1966) pointed out that a significant striving for differentiation from the "family undifferentiated ego mass" must, virtually by definition, meet an emotional response on the part of other family members, who will tend to define the differentiating behavior as bad. The family may seek a psychiatric evaluation to confirm the family pattern, reinforce the identified patient's "sick" label, and eliminate the bothersome symptoms without disrupting the underlying family dynamics. This reaction would be predictable, based on the general rule that Type I mechanisms will always be the first option. Only when Type I processes can no longer maintain homeostasis will the family consider Type II maneuvers—processes involving a shift in the reference points with respect to which the symptom functions.

A family that adapts poorly is poorly differentiated. This follows from the general premise that Type-II work is required for both adaptation and differentiation.

Mr. and Mrs. A brought four-year-old Roger to the Crisis Clinic at 2:00 A.M. The boy was wildly active: he ran frantically around the room, climbing over and under the furniture. When anyone attempted to hold him, he fought back vigorously, but made no sound and refused to speak. A physical examination, carried out with difficulty and with some hazard to the physician, revealed no abnormalities. Mr. and Mrs. A reported that Roger had become agitated the previous week and had not slept for at least two nights.

When Roger was admitted to the pediatric ward, to our surprise he promptly went to sleep. In the morning, he was pleasant, agreeable, cooperative, verbal, normally active, and friendly to other children. When the As appeared that afternoon, he resumed his wild behavior. We inferred that his behavior was a desperate request for help and could be classified as an adaptive response.

Symptoms As Maladaptive Responses

Obviously, the criteria for a maladaptive response are the opposite of those for an adaptive response. Therefore, a maladaptive response is not clearly related to environmental stress, and the new behaviors are not useful in building a healthy organism-environment relationship. In addition, there is reason to suspect that the maladaptive behaviors are not merely temporary expedients, but are becoming part of the standard behavioral repertoire (e.g., persistent fire setting with no clear antecedent or consequent conditions).

Maladaptive responses can be divided into two types: (1) those that reflect intrapsychic conflict and (2) those that reflect a core conflict in the family.

Maladaptive responses that reflect intrapsychic conflict. This type of symptom, of course, involves the classic and enormously useful concept of the neurosis—repetitive and ego-dystonic behavior that reflects an attempt to solve in the present a problem the individual was actively engaged in at an earlier time. The inference of clinically relevant conflict means that the clinician must watch for subjectively uncomfortable anxiety, unresolved grief, and depression. If the patient's symptoms do arise from intrapsychic conflict, individual psychotherapy may be the treatment of choice.

Maladaptive responses that reflect interpersonal conflict. Determining whether intrapsychic or interpersonal conflict is the primary dynamic underlying the identified patient's symptoms is absolutely essential before deciding whether the patient should be seen in individual, group, or family therapy; in another form of treatment; or not at all. We would expect the patient's symptoms to reflect a family core conflict if they are long-standing, if the developmental history of the identified patient and his family indicate that the symptoms have become a crucial component of the processes for maintaining family homeostasis, if there is evidence that the family actively supports the symptoms, if there is evidence of scapegoating, if the specific form of the symptoms seem to reflect conflicts that have been observed in one of the parents or within the marriage, and if the identified patient functions reasonably well in other environments. If the patient's symptoms improve and another family member subsequently becomes symptomatic, we have strong evidence that the patient's symptoms reflect and have helped to stabilize a conflict that has been rendered less stable by this change. Thus appropriate exploration of a family secret or a buried aspect of family mythology might lead to improved function. If the clinician suspects that interpersonal conflict is involved in the formation of the identified patient's symptoms, therapy with that social system (usually the family) may be appropriate.

Syntonicity or Dystonicity of Symptoms

Because a syntonic process pulls a system together, it will be protected and defended. A dystonic process, on the other hand, because it is experienced as expensive to the system, must be isolated or eliminated. Usually, a major objective of therapy is movement of material from the hidden syntonic realm into the visible dystonic realm. In family therapy this may require a discussion about a child's symptoms as an open expression of the hidden parental intrapsychic or intramarital conflict.

The difference between individual and family therapy is apparent. Individual therapy is impossible unless the individual experiences symptoms that are dystonic for him. In a family, however, it is entirely possible that the identified patient's symptoms are syntonic for the parents and dystonic for the child; dystonic to the parents and syntonic to the child, as in the case of a brat, or child tyrant (Barcai & Rosenthal, 1974); syntonic to the entire family while dystonic to the school, for instance. Therefore, recommendations for therapy must consider the locus of discomfort in the system! This information is frequently thrust upon us or can be obtained with a simple question such as "Who decided that you should seek psychiatric help?" or "Does anyone feel that a change is urgent?"

TREATMENT PLAN

This is a good time to point out a common clinical error: the failure to delineate clearly between evaluation and therapy. In some cases, this distinction is unimportant; occasionally, however, the clinician finds himself hopelessly confused because the contract for evaluation has merged somehow into a contract for therapy. In my experience, it is best to specify clearly to the family at the outset that the objective of the first session (and perhaps a few additional sessions) will be an evaluation. At the end of the evaluation, the family will be appraised of the clinician's impressions and recommendations.

There is no better way to gain a family's cooperation than to make it clear that the problem is so important that it needs careful evaluation and that when the evaluation is completed, the formulation will be discussed in as much detail as the family desires. Delivering an "interpretation" to a family is a supreme clinical challenge. For example, consider a case where there are biological, psychological, family, and social abnormalities; a number of conflicting diagnoses have already been obtained; and the parents are guilt-ridden about the identified patient's difficulties and angry about the rough treatment they have received from other clinicians. Our objective is to present, as clearly as possible, the contributions made by abnormality at each level and our rationale for recommending further evaluation or treatment and to accomplish all this within the context of a working alliance. Because painful feedback outside a working alliance is invariably perceived as an assault, the psychiatric clinician must work within the working alliance as meticulously as the surgeon works within the sterile and anesthetic fields. This is more easily said than done!

I find that a table of the family's major assets and liabilities (see pp. 178–179) is indispensable to accomplishing this task. If there are strong interaction between levels, these should also be discussed. Diagnosis must always be handled with care, particularly when discussing one's conclusions with an anxious parent. It is probably wise to conduct these discussions in functional terms: i.e., what do the parents need to know to manage their problems? A simple diagnostic declaration, such as "Mrs. Jones, your boy is autistic," can be brutal. If an impression is painful for a family, it may need to call or visit you again and again to reassess the situation, and a significant grieving may be involved. It may also be appropriate to warn the family that well-meaning neighbors and friends will offer newspaper clippings and magazine articles describing "cures" of one kind or another and that the child may be subjected to a variety of labels.

If *you* don't understand what's going on, say so and either refer the family elsewhere or reevaluate later. If you believe that further evaluation or therapy is not indicated, say so. And if you have encountered a new phenomenon, please write about it for the enlightenment of all!

Specific Target Problems and Interventions

Specific target problems and planned interventions on the biological, psychological, family, and social levels can be summarized in the form illustrated on pages 178 and 179. Recommendations for intervention at any level, however, necessarily assume that a significant portion of the deviation from normality can be accounted for by disorder at that level. How often do we forget to make this crucial assumption in our eagerness to proceed with our own favorite therapeutic modality? Ideally, we should make our recommendations for therapy only after due consideration of the cost/benefit ratio and possible hazards. An assault on the identified patient's self-esteem is a grim possibility in child psychiatry.

Issues related to the child. Criteria for the use of medication should include the child's perception of what that medication is for. Does he believe it is an instrument of control? Does he like himself better on or off medication?

Does the child meet the criteria for individual therapy? If so, should transference be encouraged or discouraged? Should a specific target symptom be attacked by means of desensitization? Should therapy be time limited? Would therapy stigmatize him within his family or consolidate a Sickie role to a degree that would outweigh any potential benefits of therapy? Is he accessible to therapy? Do the therapist and patient like each other?

Issues related to the family. If therapy with the identified patient is successful, is there reason to believe that another family member will become symptomatic? Is family therapy indicated at the outset? How many family members should be involved? Are members of the extended family available to therapy? Should they be included? How are the rights and feelings of *former* spouses best acknowledged?

Other issues. Should we focus primarily on the school? On the neighborhood? On referrals to other agencies?

Special Precautions

Frequently, specific urgent points merit special attention. For example, is there danger of child abuse, suicide, or serious psychosomatic illness? Are there circumstances in which the family or patient would flee abruptly from therapy? Are there idiosyncratic reactions to medications?

Are there impending legal issues? These considerations merit clear exposition at the very beginning of a written report.

Case Summaries

A careful case summary is essential and should include a brief description of the child's (1) biological predisposition, (2) developmental history, (3) current situation and (4) adaptive and maladaptive responses. The following summaries illustrate how this can be done:

> This ten-year-old Caucasian male has demonstrated a difficult temperament since birth and negativistic traits since toddlerhood. His current environment centers in a poorly defined role in his family: he has not been adopted by his mother's second husband and he has no contact with his biofather. Although there are good strengths in the family, the present symptom picture involves the rapid emergence of power struggles between the identified patient and any authority figure, especially in the context of school, school failure, assaultive behavior toward both peers and teachers, and petty theft. There is reason to suspect that the family, whose agenda seems to be extrusion of the identified patient, covertly supports these behaviors.

> This eight-year-old girl, who like her mother has suffered from a seizure disorder since birth, demonstrates depressive signs and symptoms including depressed mood; sullen, sulking behavior alternating with belligerence: and feelings of hopelessness. On the one hand, her desire for personal growth conflicts with her mother's need for a fellow sufferer. On the other hand, her self-esteem undergoes a constant battering at school because of the stigma of her frequent seizures. Therefore, it will be essential to intervene as vigorously as possible at all four levels. (1) We will seek to gain the mother's permission for the child to take medication at school and thereby insure consistent medication during the school week. (2) We will consider individual therapy with the patient to explore issues related to her self-esteem, depres-

sion, perception of her illness, etc. (3) We will make every effort to involve the mother in treatment and explore the issues related to her attempt to bind the child into a pathological relationship with respect to her seizures. (4) We will intervene at any level possible at the school: i.e., her teachers and classmates and with the administration.

Chapters 3 through 7 have attempted to summarize a vast clinical area. Although the soft spots and omissions are inevitably plentiful, I hope that the end result is a relatively comprehensive tour of a rich landscape. Many issues, of course are controversial because we know so little about behavior. The overall objective of an evaluation, of course, is a good treatment plan. Despite voluminous data our treatment plans are all-too-often poorly supported. The link between observational data and the treatment plan is, of course, the formulation. Ideally, the formulation provides so much information about the biological, developmental, and circumstantial factors in the case that the symptomatic behaviors seem almost laudable as appropriate coping maneuvers. Furthermore, the treatment plan should follow smoothly from the formulation. But unfortunately, such mastery is not common.

The next chapter describes four parameters of family function, a special tool that was mentioned only briefly earlier. This tool has proved to be so valuable that it seemed to warrant a chapter of its own.

Chapter 8

FOUR DIMENSIONS OF FAMILY FUNCTION

When viewing the family as a system, it is essential to think of it as a social *organism* that operates according to its own specific set of rules. *These rules are as much a part of the family as the individuals who compose it.* This chapter describes a clinical tool that permits us to examine some of the family rules. Developing this tool has been a fascinating task, and I hope you will find it useful.[1]

In work with families, it is essential to estimate the extent to which Commoner's first and second rules apply: (1) everything is connected to everything else, and (2) everything has to go somewhere. In Chapter 2, these rules, particularly the first one, appeared as the concept of *differentiation.* Families whose degree of differentiation is extremely low seem to defy the rules because the relationship between two or more family members is so close that the family seems to operate, not as a system in which separate elements may be identified, but as a single unit in which all pieces move together. For example, in the case of a *folie à deux,* the individuals who share a delusional system are so tightly linked that to deal with one is to deal with both. Therefore, the systems concept is not especially useful.

At the other extreme, are highly differentiated families. Members of these families experience a high degree of autonomy with respect to each other and simultaneously enjoy each other's company. In examining the lives of individual members, the rules that determine family functioning may be far less important than the rules by which individual members relate to other social systems. In the hypothetical case of a completely autonomous and self-actualizing individual who exercises free choice, the rules of the social field would not necessarily be useful when describing his behavior.

Our primary concern here is families that fall in the middle range of differentiation: i.e., Levels 2 and 3. We will be especially interested in families whose members simultaneously struggle to achieve greater distance from their families of origin and yet, because they are fearful of too great a distance, must either visit one another regularly or refuse to visit at all, lest they become enmeshed once more in the family games. As we gather more information about the specific rules of family function, it may be possible to predict which family members are at risk and, in some cases, determine the *specific hazards* they face if another family member changes. I prefer to inform families at the beginning of treatment that *therapy means change* and that we cannot predict exactly what kinds of changes may occur. Therefore, any family member who is too busy or does not believe he is involved in the symptoms may be well advised to join the family therapy sessions simply to represent his own interests as the family rewrites some important rules. In my opinion, this is not coercion; it is realistic advice.

Let me comment on two related issues. First, if we do family therapy, it is easy for us to assume that we will involve the entire family. Often, however, this is logistically impossible. Large families in which children are scattered among different schools and parents have limited resources for transportation may find that it is impossible to come together for a therapy session, especially if the sessions are scheduled during the day. If, on the other hand, we arrange evening appointments, we may impose on individuals who are fairly peripheral to the central process. Generally speaking, however, I prefer to have all family members present because those who are not essential to the core process often exert a cushioning effect. In any case, it is always useful and sometimes essential to recognize whose presence is essential and whose is a luxury. This chapter addresses this issue in operational terms.

The second issue is an extremely important one, both practically and ethically. Abrupt and even dangerous shifts occasionally occur in some families after therapy; other families make changes that result in improved functioning for everyone concerned. This chapter represents an attempt to predict which families will react in which way. To make such predictions, it is useful to examine the family system in terms of four dimensions: anxiety, capacity to change, symptom-carrier role, and power. (The power of this model will be no greater than the validity of the assumption that we are dealing with four independent variables.)

Four Dimensions Of Family Function

Anxiety

Anxiety can be defined as an unpleasant subjective sensation associated with the perception that the coping mechanisms available are inadequate to maintain homeostatis (French & Steward, 1975). It warns the organism that a deviation is not being corrected quickly enough and that the organism will be in serious trouble unless something is done—and soon! Therefore, the organism must find a way to decrease the stresses or increase the rate of correction. Anxiety may be related entirely to external circumstances, and it does not necessarily imply an unhealthy organism. Clinically, anxiety is easy to assess. We are not interested here in "masked" anxiety but in an apparent, subjectively uncomfortable state that may function as a motivating force. Anxiety is the signal that Type I processes are inadequate.

Capacity for Change

Our second parameter, the capacity for change, is the ability to relinquish previously useful reference points with respect to which homeostatis was maintained and to adopt new ones that are more in line with current reality. It is identical to the capacity to carry out Type II processes (accommodation, or a shift in the family reference system) and is closely related to the parameter of *differentiation.* Because assessing a family's capacity to change is often difficult, the clinician must have a fair amount of exposure to the family. In some cases, clues can be obtained from the life histories of individual members; in others, there is ample evidence of repetitive, painful life situations and little or no change. Observing family members in the office may also provide clues. For example, how do they respond to interpretations, suggestions, and so forth?

Symptom-carrier Role

Here we are concerned with the probability that the role of symptom carrier will be applied to a specific individual. We are also concerned with the rigidity of the role as expressed in the following statement: "*Of course* I know that Johnny did it, even though I didn't see him. He always does those sorts of things." In the literature, this role has been called scapegoating, and it is easy to assess clinically. The family may literally walk in the door announcing: "Here is the family member responsible for all our troubles!" If this role seems relatively rigid, another person who is initially less conspicuous is probably just as important in this parameter. Is there someone in the family who is revered by all and can do no wrong? (For a general discussion of this type of analysis see Laughlin & D'Aquili, 1974.) Because individuals will have differing opinions concerning which member is the symptom carrier, it is useful to specify the observer. (This may apply in any of the four parameters, of course, but it is especially applicable here.) Often a system in crisis will be divided, with each part seeking to scapegoat the other.

Power

Power is defined as the ability to distribute individuals within the three-dimensional space generated by the first three parameters. That is, if one member of a social system decides (1) who will be anxious, (2) who will be expected to accommodate to change while others remain where they are and simply assimilate, and (3) who will be tagged as the symptom carrier when the going gets rough, that member does indeed wield power!

Power is difficult to estimate clinically, and the picture is often confused (Cartwright, 1959). One family member (usually the identified patient) *appears* to wield power in the family, while another family member, usually a parent, determines the course of events through subtle but powerful manipulation of roles. Therefore, be extremely suspicious if the individual who is labeled symptom-carrier also seems to rank high in power. This configuration is unlikely. If it appears, make certain that a parent is not using the scapegoat to mask his own power.

Because a four-dimensional space is impossible to visualize, I use a chart, placing each family member in each horizontal column from lowest on the left to highest on the right. This enables me to rank family members along each dimension. Let's look at two examples: the Jones family and the Edwards family.

CASE STUDIES

The Jones Family

Mr. and Mrs. Jones have requested an evaluation of their ten-year-old son, Eddie, who is in a program for the educationally handicapped at school. Because Eddie functions poorly, even in this special environment, his parents suspect that he is mentally retarded.

Mr. Jones has been employed intermittently for the past few years, and the family has been in severe financial difficulty. Mrs. Jones's mother, who lives nearby, helps the family in a variety of ways. Although she does not come to the clinic, her daughter describes her as "the sweetest, most lovable person you ever saw." The grandmother attends church frequently and busies herself in a variety of helpful activities.[2] Her husband died some years ago as a result of complications related to alcoholism. Mr. Jones's relatives live in a distant state and he rarely sees them. He describes his mother as "a hard woman, with too many kids" and his father as "pretty much a drifter who came by and took care of us when there was work in town." The identified patient is the youngest of four children; the parents report that they have had few problems with the other children. Their 19-year-old son has been in the Marines for a year and is apparently functioning satisfactorily. Their 18-year-old daughter married her high school sweetheart six months ago "to get away from all the bickering and fighting," and their 12-year-old daughter is apparently asymptomatic.

Eddie presents no chief complaint. He understands that he is to have tests but believes that his schoolwork is satisfactory. His facial expression indicates anxiety, and his answers to questions are brief. He sits restlessly in his chair, ignoring the toys on the shelf, and fidgets and squirms, constantly biting and picking at his fingernails.

Mr. and Mrs. Jones present a different picture. Mrs. Jones is agitated and frequently snaps at Eddie: "Eddie! Sit up and answer the doctor's question!" Mr. Jones glowers in agreement. Mrs. Jones weeps periodically as she describes her frustration about Eddie's school performance and her husband's drinking problem. At this, Mr. Jones abruptly becomes angry and bellows: "Now, you shut up. We're here to talk about Eddie's tests!" But Mrs. Jones continues to discuss his drinking, while Mr. Jones mutters occasionally in disagreement. During this exchange, Eddie slouches in his chair, stares vacantly at his feet, and picks at his fingernails. Mrs. Jones crying more loudly, says that she divorced her first husband because he drank heavily and beat her periodically. She then married Mr. Jones because he was "a steady fellow and a good provider," but he has turned out to be just like her first husband.

We ask more about the family. "Is there anyone else who lives in the area or is important to the family?" No. Mrs. Jones's two older sisters live in a neighboring state. "Is there anyone whose good will you would not dare to lose, or whose advice you would never want to ignore?" Mrs. Jones shakes her head, but Mr. Jones, seeing his opportunity to counterattack, says: "Your mother! Hell, you run to her for everything." Mrs. Jones replies, "No, Ed, that isn't what the doctor means." We then ask who actually runs things in the family. Eddie smiles slightly and mumbles "Grandma." His father nods in agreement, while Mrs. Jones replies: "Well, but she always *helps* us. That isn't what you mean, is it?"

Eddie's teacher, contacted with the family's permission, describes him as disruptive and inattentive in class. He has few friends, and children usually try to avoid him.

Let's look at the Jones family in terms of our four-place table. First, all members of the family system must be included. It is easiest to begin with the extremely high and extremely low positions. Mrs. Jones ranks high in terms of anxiety; Mr. Jones and Eddie fall in the intermediate range. With the family's permission, we call Mrs. Jones's mother, who says she is very concerned about Eddie and always has been. In fact, as much as she loves them all, he is her favorite grandchild. She certainly hopes the doctor can straighten out his teachers. They aren't very nice to Eddie; what he needs is a little understanding. She is not interested in coming to the clinic; why would she come in to talk to the doctor about Eddie. She's very busy around the house, at church, and with her children. She is careful not to interfere, of course, but she's happy to help out whenever she can. She has no idea who makes the decisions in the family? Mr. Jones should, of course, but then he can hardly be called the head of the household since he drinks so much. What does all this have to do with Eddie's tests anyway? Based on what we know so far, Eddie's grandmother does not rank in anxiety. In fact, she seems comfortable with herself and her life and attributes the difficulties of others to their lack of temperance of one kind or another.

Who has the capacity to change? There is no clear history of accommodation on anyone's part. Mrs. Jones is now in her second marriage, which seems similar to the first. Her capacity to change is probably not high. Mr. Jones seems to handle life stress by drinking. We do not know enough yet about Eddie. Eddie's grandmother certainly is not motivated to change the current situation, and his brother and sisters are unknown entities at this point.

In the column labeled symptom-carrier role, Eddie ranks high; his father is occasionally tagged as symptom carrier. Mrs. Jones's position is unclear. Because Eddie's grandmother seems beyond reproach, she ranks extremely low in this column.

Who wields the power in this family? Eddie seems to rank extremely low in terms of ability to determine the roles of family members. Mrs. and Mr. Jones apparently are engaged in a power struggle; Mrs. Jones won the bout in the office. We suspect that Mr. Jones's drinking may be related to this process. We ask who buys the liquor. Eddie reports that "Mama brings it home with the groceries." Mrs. Jones tearfully explains. "If I don't, he just goes and gets it himself anyway, and he gets in such a mean, ugly mood. I don't like for him to hit me." All the evidence indicates that Eddie's grandmother wields more power in the family than anyone else.

We can now translate these inferences to the table, using the following designations: Eddie (I.P.), Mrs. Jones (M), Mr. Jones (F), and the grandmother (Gm). This gives us the following configuration:

Dimension	Low	High
Anxiety	Gm, I.P., F	M
Capacity to change	F? M?	
Symptom-carrier role	Gm, F, M	I.P.
Power	I.P., F, M,	Gm

We have all seen families such as this, and we are familiar with the different courses they can take over time. All family members can remain the same or they can improve. Or some can improve while others become worse. Our concern is the chronicity of family patterns. In the Jones family, the history of alcoholism, Eddie's special place as the youngest child, and the relationship between Eddie's parents and his grandmother indicate a family-syntonic problem. That is, the family structure may involve the

Game of Rescue (see Berne, 1964). If so, the family requires one rescuer. Eddie is a vulnerable candidate for this role because he is the youngest child, grandmother's favorite, male (the only functional male in the family, since Eddie's older brother, has left home), and a failure in school. Eddie's difficulties, although distressing to him and his family, are an important part of the family structure. The recent increase in Mr. Jones's drinking raises the possibility that the family needs more activity in the area of rescue at this point. The degree to which family roles are fixed cannot be estimated with certainty, but alcoholism in at least two generations argues for fairly rigid roles. The clinical impact of these issues is that any improvement in Eddie's functioning may meet with strong covert resistance from his family and that major improvement may be followed by a significant amount of deterioration in another family member.

When we deferred the family's request for extensive psychological testing pending clarification of other issues, Eddie's father withdrew, denouncing us as "a bunch of damn Freudians." When we suggested that Eddie might benefit from individual therapy, Mrs. Jones agreed and talked to his therapist before each session. She anticipated our suggestion that she might benefit from therapy by denying that her problems merited a therapist's attention. Eddie's older sisters refused to come to the clinic, and Mr. and Mrs. Jones supported their decision.

Eddie improved. His vision, which we discovered poor, was corrected with glasses, and his school work and relationships with classmates immediately improved. He developed a good relationship with the therapist and actively took part in play therapy. After one month of therapy, Mrs. Jones announced that Eddie was "a little more likeable in some ways, but he's getting to be hyperactive and sassy." She was particularly concerned because he was "disrespectful" to his grandmother occasionally.

Eddie failed to report for his eighth session. Although Mrs. Jones expressed regret about failing to call us, but she had been busy because her mother had been ill. Three weeks later, when Eddie reappeared at the clinic, his mother said he was "acting worse than ever" and suggested that medication might "calm him down." Rather than engage the therapist in play or conversation, Eddie wandered listlessly about the playroom, saying little and avoiding questions. Both he and the therapist were relieved when the session was over.

Three days later Mrs. Jones called to say that she could not bring Eddie in "for a while." Her mother was ill again and required daily care—and anyway, the school did not complain about him any more. When we called four weeks later, the family situation was about the same. Two months later, another call revealed that Eddie was "about the same" at school; his grandmother had recovered from a vague, lingering illness; and the family was not interested in coming back to the clinic.

Based on the family history of alcoholism, Mrs. Jones's two marriages, and the family's dependence on her mother, we can rank the family's degree of differentiation at Level 2. In other words, we can assume that these four individuals form a system in which, to a significant extent, everything is connected to everything else and everything has to go somewhere.

Let's look at Eddie in terms of the four-place table. Based on his improved performance at school and in the playroom, we can infer that his anxiety has decreased. Furthermore the fact that he gets along better at school is making it increasingly difficult for the family to view him as the symptom carrier and indicates that he is capable of changing his life to some extent. Based on Mrs. Jones's complaint that Eddie is becoming "sassy and disrespectful," we can infer that he is striving for more power in the family. These changes can be noted as follows:

Dimension	Low	High
Anxiety	← I.P.	
Capacity to change	I.P. →	
Symptom-carrier role		← I.P.
Power	I.P. →	

Now, if we assume that everything is connected to everything else and everything has to go somewhere, we can conclude that Eddie's changes will require other family members to change. The table enables us to predict, with only an empirical justification, that the family will tend to balance itself somewhere around a midline. That is, if someone ranks low in one column, the family will have to add "weight" on the other side of the midline. Similarly, we can predict that individual family members will tend to balance around the midline. If Eddie's role as symptom carrier is less rigid and his power has increased, how will balance be reestablished? The grandmother is most vulnerable because her positions are the most extreme; thus the balance would be reestablished by raising her rank as symptom carrier and reducing her power—and automatically increasing her anxiety:

Dimension	Low	High
Anxiety	Gm →	
Capacity to change	Gm? →	
Symptom-carrier role	Gm →	I.P.
Power	I.P.	← Gm

There are two lines of evidence for this shift. One, the grandmother became ill when Eddie improved: i.e., her illness may have been related to stress caused by a shift in the family role structure.[3] Two, Mrs. Jones reported that Eddie was becoming disrespectful to his grandmother. This might represent an effort on Eddie's part to move his grandmother up in the symptom-carrier column: i.e., he might be asking her to take her turn in the hot seat. In restrospect, then, the four-place table "explains" our clinical observations.

What other configurations come to mind? An obvious one is that Mr. Jones might drink more and work less. This behavior would represent a trade off between Eddie and his father: i.e., if Eddie improves, another individual's functioning must deteriorate. The third possibility is similar to the first: no change would occur in the family's essential rules; only the names of individuals filling the specific roles would change. In other words, the grandmother's position would not be challenged. That is, the family would not make a Type II change; it would confine itself to Type I maneuvers alone and leave the basic role structure in tact.

A healthier family would make a series of turnovers and in the process would become more flexible, achieve greater degrees of freedom, and reduce its symptoms. In other words, *all* members might benefit from change.

Eddie's family presented a typical set of configurations: the grandmother ranked low in terms of anxiety and the role of symptom carrier and high in power. Eddie's level of anxiety was intermediate and his capacity for change was unclear; he ranked high as symptom carrier and low in power. Using the designations, L = low, H = high, M = medium, and ? = unclear, and maintaining a rigid ordering of our four parameters—i.e., (1) anxiety, (2) capacity for change, (3) symptom carrier, and (4) power, the grandmother is LLLH and Eddie is MMHL. (Because of its peculiar shape, the LLLH profile is called the "hockey stick." The individual with a hockey-stick profile wields an enormous amount of power.) Mrs. Jones is HLMH. Her configuration is an interesting one because she simultaneously ranks high in anxiety and wields significant power in the family. Her life course indicates a limited capacity for change. This HLMH configuration is common among individuals diagnosed as "personality disorder, masochistic type." Obviously, a person who ranks high in both anxiety and power for a long time will be described as masochistic. This description is appropriate if it can be established that the individual uses power to maintain himself in a high-anxiety position.

The LLLH (grandmother), MMHL (Eddie), and HLMH (Mrs. Jones) configurations are extremely common and will appear throughout this discussion. Therefore, a clear impression of the type of clinical picture they represent is useful.

Eddie's therapy and improved vision moved him into a midline configuration, and we can speculate that linkages within the family operated in such a way that his grandmother's anxiety concomitantly increased. The grandmother's *shift from LLLH to HLHH is extremely important: if this transition cannot be tolerated, the case will be lost!* In this case, Eddie's therapy was interrupted because Mrs. Jones invested her energy in her mother's illness. If a family resists further therapy despite the presence of symptoms, if there is reason to believe that a shift in one member's functioning is linked to a shift in another's—particularly if improvement in one is followed by deterioration in another—and if there are no important extenuating circumstances, we can conclude that the family roles are rigid and that the family has concluded that additional improvement in the identified patient is not worth the risks. *This decision must be respected!* The family may be saying: "We have exhausted Type I maneuvers, and further change will require a Type II maneuver of some sort. We don't know what this will be—a serious illness, a divorce, or some other catastrophe. We are not willing to take this risk." Everyone might improve too, but many troubled families apparently believe that this is unlikely.

The Edwards Family

Mr. and Mrs. Edwards were directed by the juvenile court to seek a psychiatric evaluation of their 14-year-old daughter, Joan. The girl had been a truant from school and had stayed out all night with friends; she had also been drinking and stealing money from her mother and stepfather.

Joan was well dressed and seemed older than her years. She was annoyed about having to "see a dumb shrink" and viewed her behavior as appropriate. Mrs. Edwards cried and seemed to feel hopeless. She blamed herself for Joan's behavior, but had no clear idea about what she could have done differently.

A brief developmental history provided the following information: Joan had always been "headstrong." Mrs. Edwards had divorced Joan's father when Joan was two and "got into the bad habit of buying Joan off to stop her temper tantrums." Things generally went well when Joan had her way, but she demanded a high price for her cooperation. Joan's stepfather usually agreed with his wife and offered no opinions of his own.

We asked who held power in the family. Joan immediately replied "I do" as though the answer was obvious. Mrs. Edwards looked startled, but her husband said "I guess she's right, honey."

The positions of Joan and her mother in the four-dimensional table are clear. Joan views the entire system, including the clinican and the court, as symptomatic, while the court views things the other way around. Mr. Edward's position is not clear. Joan holds the same position that Eddie's grandmother held; Mrs. Edwards position is similar to Eddie's, but she seems more anxious.

This family configuration is common and probably represents the majority of cases in some agencies. Barcai

Dimension	Low		High
Anxiety	Joan		Mother
Capacity to change	Joan?	Mother?	
Symptom-carrier role	(Joan's view) Joan		Mother
	(Mother's view) Mother		Joan
Power		Mother Joan	

and Rosenthal (1974) call it the "tyrannical child" configuration and claim that extrusion of the child, who may then reenter the family only under the family's terms, is the best treatment in some cases. They point out, however, that this maneuver may precipitate a major crisis.

Joan's case was a difficult one. The parents finally recognized after months of counseling that they were afraid of Joan and that the situation would change only if they were to set limits for her. When Mrs. Edward's fears were explored, she tearfully said that she "absolutely could not bear to hurt her baby any more than she had already." The implications of the alternative she had chosen, however, were clear. As her parents began to impose limits, Joan carried out a series of increasingly flagrant and dangerous testing maneuvers, while her stepfather became an increasingly competent parent. A key component of this process was the parents' ability to stand together on important issues.[4]

The turning point occurred on a weekend, when Joan and some friends took the family car without permission and returned at dawn. Mr. Edwards subsequently reported: "I don't know if I should have done it, but, what I did was —Well, in plain language, I paddled her 14-year-old ass." In response Joan retreated to her room and announced that she would never go to school again. Her parents insisted that she return to school and the situation was a stand-off. The therapist heard about the incident the following Monday morning and set up an appointment for the three of them that day. At this point, the family's configuration was as follows:

Dimension	Low		High
Anxiety			Joan Parents
Capacity to change		Joan	Parents
Symptom-carrier role	(Joan's view) Joan		Parents
	(Parents'view)	Parents	Joan
Power		Joan	Parents

An active power struggle was obviously in progress. This configuration is so important that it warrants discussion. I call it "Ping-pong" or "Warfare," depending on the intensity of the interaction. Both parties are anxious, there is an active power struggle, each party tries to avoid making a major accommodative change, and each is convinced that [s]he is right and the other is wrong. This configuration follows naturally from a confrontation between an LLLH and an HLHL and represents a common transient, intermediate phase. A healthy family will experiment with this configuration briefly, cushioning the interaction with horseplay and humor. Thus for adults as well as children, play makes possible a reversible examination of a set of alternatives that would be too frightening to consider if it led to an *irreversible* transition to an alternate configuration. The Ping-pong combination is healthy as a short-lived intermediate form that indicates a transition. But if chronic, the Ping-pong configuration spells trouble! If the intensity of interaction is low, the two contending parties (e.g., a married couple) may engage for years in a subtle but powerful and corrosive conflict. The term Ping-pong is appropriate because the children in these situations are literally bounced back and forth as each parent seeks to support his perception that his spouse is the symptom carrier. Do not be deceived by the calm front these couples present to the world. If sociocultural factors forbid the outward display of displeasure or aggression, the most subtle kinds of interaction may be as effective as a well-flung plate would be in a different subculture. In general, variable and content-appropriate affect indicates a flexible system. Fixed affect, *including fixed cheerfulness or fixed evenness,* may indicate that a tight game is being played for high stakes.

If extremely intense this game becomes Warfare. Couples who play this game crash into homicide, suicide, psychosis, pregnancy, abortion, and major decisions, tran-

sitions, and disasters of all kinds. Chronic warfare is probably identical to the schism described by Lidz, Cornelison,
Fleck & Terry (1957) in which couples express their deep
bond by fighting. The traumatic effect on children is enormous, and paranoia in various forms is common among
children of these families.

Let's return to Joan. Joan was finally willing to speak
to a therapist alone, and a subsequent conjoint session with
the entire family was possible. During the conjoint session,
we explored the imbalance of power that had existed in the
family and the high price that all family members had paid
to maintain it. It was now clear that Joan, the tyrant, feared
that a shift in the family power structure would put her in
the dungeon. At the end of the session, the school issue was
unresolved, and both Joan and her parents were determined to have things their way.

Two days later, the family's demeanor was strikingly
different—all three were more relaxed. Mrs. Edwards announced: "We don't know who won." Joan burst into
laughter. Her mother continued: "On the way home Joan
said, 'OK, I've made up my mind, and nothing you can say
will change me.' We were ready for the worst. Then Joan
said 'I'm going back to school!' " At this point, Joan broke
into gales of laughter.

This story has a happy ending. Although similar struggles subsequently occurred, they were progressively less
severe. Six months later, Joan had a new circle of friends
and the family was stable. No new dysfunction appeared in
any family member. Joan summed it up this way: "We have
a family now." The spanking had not represented a simple
turnover, in which the parents would have become LLLH
and forced Joan into an HLHL configuration. The crisis
was adaptive because it involved a shift of all positions in
the family role structure. As a result, the family gained in
both balance and flexibility.

USE OF THE FOUR-DIMENSIONAL MODEL

It is now possible to discuss some general points related to the use of the four-dimensional table. But first, it is important to point out again the three most common configurations: the hockey stick, the zig-zag, and the masochist.

The hockey stick, or LLLH configuration, typified by Eddie's grandmother (and by Joan before treatment therapy), is illustrated in the following table:

Dimension	Low	High
Anxiety	X	
Capacity to change	X	
Symptom-carrier role	X	
Power		X

The scapegoat or "patient" typically has the a zig-zag configuration (HLHL): i.e., he ranks high in anxiety, low or medium in capacity to change, high or superhigh as the symptom carrier, and low in power. The following table illustrates his profile:

Dimension	Low	High
Anxiety		X
Capacity to change	X	
Symptom-carrier role		X
Power	X	

The masochist, or HLMH configuration is all too familiar to clinicians. This individual ranks high in both anxiety and power, his endless misery from childhood through adulthood demonstrates a minimal capacity to change, and yet he ranks high in terms of power to determine family roles:

Dimension	Low	High
Anxiety		X
Capacity to change	X	
Symptom-carrier role	X	
Power		X

A few family members usually "float" somewhere in the middle along all four dimensions. Their positions may be visible only during a crisis, if at all.

Heuristic Rules

The model presented here is at best prescientific. We have not yet reached the stage of crisp, testable hypotheses. The following heuristic rules, however, are clinically useful and may lead to testing of hypotheses:

1. Healthy systems permit reversible shifts in roles as a function of stress; an unhealthy system is role-rigid. Therefore, if we see evidence that family members have maintained one configuration for a long time, even if that configuration falls in the midline of the table, we are probably dealing with a fixed system which handles stress poorly, is filled with hidden balance bargains, and tends to use scapegoating extensively during crises. The family members may exchange roles, but the basic structure remains constant. These families are customarily described in somewhat derogatory terms and in a derogatory tone. An alternative is to view the repetition of patterns from one generation to the next as loyalty among people whose loyalty takes an all-or-none form.

2. The family must maintain balance. Therefore, if an individual shifts his position along any of the four dimensions, a compensatory shift must occur somewhere else in the system. This generalization applies *only* in families that do not rank extremely high in differentiation.

3. Assuming a low-stress environment, members of healthy families usually cluster around the mid-line and exchange roles periodically. An unhealthy system will suffer extreme displacements.

4. A family will usually claim that the identified patient (or anyone who ranks highest in the symptom-carrier column) wields the most power. Therefore, the clinician must distinguish carefully between the power to act up and the power to determine role structure. If the same person appears at the high end of both the symptom carrier and power columns, someone is probably pulling the wool over your eyes. And that someone is probably the one who actually wields the power!

5. As therapy proceeds, the family will experiment with different configurations. This experimentation is the logical result of rules 1 and 3. *For significant structural change to occur, the family must be willing to experiment with at least one full rotation of configurations.* In other words, everyone must take his turn on the hotseat at least once. Once again, preoperational thought exerts a decisive influence: if the person in power cannot imagine this as a *reversible* process, he perceives the price of change as enormously high! Who among us would readily exchange a throne for a dungeon, even to rescue someone we love and put him on the throne? (And if we did so, would we be labeled a masochist?)

6. As a family moves from one configuration to another, it will experience a transient increase in disorder. This rule seems to apply across the board—from chemical and physical systems to large social systems. Consequently, if the clinician decides to precipitate a crisis, he must anticipate the possible consequences.

7. The magnitude of the disorder during a crisis usually is inversely proportional to the family's level of differentiation. Here again, we see a relationship between Bowen's concept of differentiation (1966), the Type II

changes discussed in Chapter 1, and Commoner's rules (1971) that everything is connected to everything else and everything must go somewhere. A poorly differentiated family cannot carry out Type II processes easily, and Commoner's two system rules apply rigidly. The family may avoid change for a long period, then change abruptly and violently. The LLLH-HLHL pair will go through an intermediate transitional phase where both are anxious and engaged in an active power struggle. If the family's degree of differentiation is low, this phase may be dangerous for the system. The importance of assessing the family's capacity for change cannot be overemphasized. When a clinician is in trouble, he has almost always *overestimated* the capacity of an individual or family to change. The family will respond with a behavioral plea for him to recognize how difficult and frightening Type II processes can be.

8. A request for help usually implies that an overt or covert power struggle is going on somewhere in the system. Therefore, we can designate the right half of the power column as the power corner because power struggles usually occur there. A common example would involve a confrontation between an LLLH and an HLHL. To reduce his own anxiety, the HLHL may challenge the LLLH in some way. Based on the parameters outlined in Rule 7, this may be a fairly desperate move (even a revolution or armed coup). The LLLH individual immediately becomes anxious, his capacity to change is tested, and he tends to be labeled scapegoat if the challenging scapegoat achieves enough power to cast him into that role.

9. For change to occur, all four parameters—anxiety, capacity to change, symptom-carrier role, and power must be adequately represented. If the level of any one is too low, therapy will proceed slowly. If anxiety is low, there will be little motivation to change. If there is no capacity to change, obviously there will be no change. If there is no symptom carrier, the family will remain passive or complain

about the people "out there." And if there is no power to readjust major life patterns, no patterns will be changed. Because of this rule, the right-hand third or so of the area included in the four columns is designated as the therapy field.

A Practical Problem

It is now possible to address our first general question again: if change is indicated, who should be involved? We can now reply that ideally, therapy should involve everyone who appears in the therapy field, even if in only one parameter. For example, in the Jones family, therapy will necessarily affect and be affected by, and therefore should ideally involve Mrs. Jones (anxiety), Eddie (symptom carrier), and the grandmother (Power). Mr. Jones is a floater, i.e., his role is unclear. Furthermore, the four-dimensional table predicts that the case will be limited by the family's capacity to change—or more precisely, by the person in power's capacity to change (the grandmother in this case). Retrospective predictions are always safe, so we can safely predict that the case will run afoul of the grandmother's limited capacity to change. Indeed, she developed a vague illness, which required her daughter's energy and made further therapy for Eddie impossible. As indicated earlier, the two processes may have been linked.

In the case of the Edwards family, the therapy field initially included Mrs. Edwards and Joan. Joan alone presented no obvious route to therapy because she was not anxious in a clinically useful way and because she wielded enough power to fend off anxiety. Mrs Edwards alone was a reasonable candidate. The table predicts a power struggle between Joan and her mother, the outcome of which depends on Mrs. Edward's capacity to change. The increase in Mr. Edward's power—together with the couple's new-found ability to maintain a coherent position—was obviously the decisive factor. The change in the family occurred as first Mrs. Edwards and then Mr. Edwards made significant changes.

This is a good time to comment on what McDermott and Char (1974) called the "undeclared war between child and family therapy." Neither individual nor family therapy should be used blindly or as the method of choice in every case. Sometimes the therapy field includes a group of reasonably accessible individuals whose simultaneous presence in therapy (whether in parallel or together is a tangential point) generates optimal progress. If individuals who appear in the therapy field are inaccessible, then several outcomes are possible. If changes do occur, particularly if the family is not highly differentiated, all individuals who appear in the therapy field will impinge on and will themselves be influenced by the therapy in one way or another. The four-dimensional table should provide some clues about what kinds of influences may arise and from where. In long-term therapy, when analysis of the transference is the primary focus, the transference will "replace" the missing individual or individuals in the form of transference projection.

Transitions

So far, I have alluded to several transitions. We may now make them explicit. First, there is the transition that occurs when an LLLH individual experiences increasing anxiety. If he is not willing to give up some of his power, become a scapegoat, or change, the situation is a highly conflicted one. The illness of Eddie's grandmother may reflect a process of this type. This transition has the following appearance:

Dimension	Low	High
Anxiety	G →	
Capacity to change	G →	
Symptom-carrier role	G →	
Power		← G

Dimension	Low		High
Anxiety	J	⌒⤫⌒	M
Capacity to change	J ⟵²M⟶²		
Symptom-carrier role	J	⌒⤫⌒	M
Power	M ⤫ J		

Second is the transition called family turnover, which was discussed in the context of the Edwards family. This phase occurs when LLLH and HLHL trade places and may cause considerable turbulence. During family turnover, the table will look like the following:

The question marks over the arrows indicate an increase in the capacity to change in both LLLH (Joan) and HLHL (her mother) if their crisis is an adaptive one and if they are less extreme in their positions and less rigid than before. However, if they cannot change, they only change positions. If the system is maladaptive, the distortions may be more extreme and the system may become more rigid than before. A couple with chronic, rigidly fixed LLLH and HLHL positions may fit the pattern of marital skew described by Lidz et al. (1957).

An extremely important state is one in which two people hold the HLLH configuration and are engaged in an active power struggle. Each seeks to decrease his anxiety and avoid the symptom-carrier role and each views the other as symptomatic. Designating the observer in parentheses and dividing the symptom-carrier column accordingly gives us the following configuration:

Dimension	Low	High
Anxiety		X Y
Capacity to change	Y X	
Symptom-carrier role	(X) X	Y
	(Y) Y	
Power		X Y

This configuration sometimes occurs briefly during a turnover. But if neither party will change, accept the scapegoat (HLHL) configuration, or leave the system, the result is Warfare. In some cases, the two parties involved are at extreme odds; threats of homicide and suicide are commonplace and may be carried out. Paranoia or paranoid schizophrenia is often diagnosed in families where this configuration is chronic. The old clinical rule that an unstable dyad soon becomes a triad is relevant here. Often, a couple in this configuration play Ping-pong, using the identified patient as the ball. If the process does not consume all the system's energy, one contesting party may resort to virtually any coping maneuver to maintain the balance of power. Although these maneuvers generate fireworks in some subcultures and are carried out *sotto voce* in others, the results are always devastating. The family that handles crises by throwing plates is clinically difficult in many ways, but its rules can be examined relatively easy. The impeccably polished upper-class family may be more pleasant to work with, but evaluation can be enormously challenging since crucial exchanges between the HLLH and HLLH are carried out through subtle innuendoes. Examples of subtle warfare are ubiquitous among professionals of all kinds, military men, missionaries, and artists: "We agree, of course, dear, that X is an unassailably worthy cause. I am going to do X. You cannot question my motivations; to do so would challenge the very rules of our marriage. In doing X, I am above criticism because we have agreed that it is *always* good to [save lives, protect the country, save souls, pursue my Muse, . . .]." This situation is similar to what Lidz et al. (1957) called marital schism, where a couple stay together despite extensive overt hostility.

A Common Clinical Error

The four-dimensional table helps us to understand the reasons for a common clinical error-overidentification with one's patient. According to the table, the process is as follows: The identified patient (HLHL configuration) is seen in individual therapy. The parents or parent (LLLH configuration) are either seen by another clinician in the context of family therapy or not seen at all. Traditionally, a psychiatrist sees the identified patient while a social worker sees the parents. As the family system approaches a crisis, the social worker has the most difficult job—but I have already stated my feelings about this in the Preface. In any case, the psychiatrist and social worker identify with their respective clients and at some point have the following conversation: *Psychiatrist.* "Why don't you do something to protect my kid from those terrible people?" *Social worker.* "Why don't *you* do something to protect my parents from that nasty little kid you're supposed to be curing?"

Both parties then indulge in subtle forms of misbehavior, such as skipping or arriving late for meetings that were scheduled to "straighten out the whole problem," setting up family members to act out the therapists' desires, and so on. The two therapists are usually enacting a struggle that mirrors to a large degree the one going on in the family. This, of course, may be an opportunity for the two of them (occasionally with the help of a "super therapist") to resolve their own dispute and, in the process, learn how to help the family.

This situation is equally likely to arise during conjoint family therapy. The therapist identifies with the HLHL and seeks to protect him. If change occurs, an LLLH family member will sooner or later begin to feel the pressure. The more pitiful the HLHL's plight and the more rigid the family, the more severe will be the LLLH's plight during therapy and the greater the danger of a complete turnover (rather than a more adaptive shift toward the midline) and the greater the therapist's temptation to say, in one way or another, as the LLLH becomes anxious: "Good enough for you, you mean old so-and-so. You've been making the life of my poor little friend, the scapegoat, miserable! If you think *this* is bad, wait til you see what's coming next!" Often, however, the family does not stay to find out. At some point, it begins to experience a transition into the Warfare configuration, which is often heralded by subdivision of the symptom-carrier column as the identified patient becomes strong enough to challenge his role as scapegoat and attempts to share it with others. If the family turns to the therapist for help and hears "Just you wait for what's coming next," it will probably discontinue therapy. At that point, the therapist can say: "They weren't motivated. Just as things began to improve, they quit."

Please consider the following working hypothesis carefully: The reason the LLLH is so ornery is precisely because he has, locked up in his tender insides, his own miserable scapegoat. He perceives himself as seriously threatened and perceives the family configuration as essential to his well-being. As therapy proceeds, the LLLH fears (perhaps quite realistically, particularly if he is a member of a poorly differentiated family) that he will be forced willy-nilly into the HLHL configuration. Because a Type II change forced on one by external factors is difficult in the best of circumstances, is it any wonder that competent therapy is resisted so frequently?

Although it is often difficult to treat an HLHL identified patient, the problems are usually straightforward clinical ones. *Identifying and adopting a supportive stance toward the LLLH individual is usually the core of the case.* It is easy to invest energy in the well-being of a suffering, scapegoated, HLHL patient. But to identify and work skillfully and effectively with the LLLH member of the family takes a real clinician!

NOTES

1. This chapter is a modified version of a paper by A. P. French and B. Guidera titled "The family as a system in four dimensions: A theoretical model," which was presented at the American Academy of Child Psychiatry, San Francisco, California, 1974.
2. Although the role of religion in families is often a powerful one, we are specifically concerned with the interpersonal use of religious activity rather than with religious belief or practice per se. Destructive interpersonal power can be derived from passionate involvement in any activity, including child psychiatry.
3. Causality in this case would be difficult to demonstrate rigorously. Nevertheless, a new dysfunction commonly appears in one family member when another member improves. Perhaps genuine hypothesis testing will be possible in this area in the future.
4. In these cases, one parent's efforts to set limits are almost invariably sabotaged by the other, who rescues the child from the stress created by the imposition of limits. Therefore, one important facet of therapy is to help the parents find a common ground before they attempt to set limits. This can be difficult if the parents never agree on anything.

Chapter 9

TOOLS FOR DAILY USE

Chapters 3 through 7 provided a comprehensive survey of how to attack a child-family problem. We must now attack a different problem: What small set of cognitive tools is useful in day-to-day practice? And how do we maximize both their usefulness and problem-solving power?

Each clinician must solve this problem for himself. In my opinion, one should first examine a wide range of tools by examining a few cases in detail, using every piece of information in Chapters 3 through 7, and then settle on a few tools for daily use.

My own tool kit consists of an abbreviated outline consisting of (1) identifying data, (2) a summary of the clinical problem, (3) temperamental type, (4) developmental history, (5) family tree, (6) degree of differentiation, (7) assessment of family dynamics by means of the four-place table described in the previous chapter, and, of course, (8) clinical observations. These tools should permit the development of a formulation involving biological, developmen-

239

tal, and current circumstantial factors and coping mechanisms; a discussion of diagnostic possibilities (using GAP Report No 62); and a problem-plan list. The following case examples will illustrate how they can be used:

LOWELL ROLLA

Lowell Rolla, age 4½, came to our attention when his mother called the clinic in a state of distress. According to the intake sheet, Lowell lived with his mother and stepfather. His mother's chief complaint was: "He's just wild. He won't mind. He beats up on his brother and doesn't care. He might have to be put away somewhere." We called Mrs. Rolla to confirm the appointment and asked whether the situation was an emergency. "Well, no, I guess not. I was just a little hysterical when I called because Lowell had just beat up on his brother again. I don't know if I should come in. Will it help?" An appointment was scheduled for that week, and we asked if Mr. Rolla would come in. "Well, of course he works, and I don't think he'd be interested in talking to a psychiatrist." Mrs. Rolla and her son arrived on time for their appointment.

We observed the mother and son in the waiting room. Mrs. Rolla, a young, well-dressed, neatly groomed young woman, sat reading a magazine. Lowell sat on the same couch, approximately three feet away from her, swinging his feet. Twice within a few minutes, he reached over to touch his mother's arm, apparently to gain her attention. She responded with what appeared to be exasperation; her general manner indicated an attitude of "What now?" She maintained eye contact with Lowell only fleetingly and answered his questions with a minimum of words. When invited into the office, Lowell asked "Are you the doctor?" and Mrs. Rolla smiled and put away the magazine. Lowell ran immediately to the drinking fountain. His mother

called after him, "Lowell, no!" He ignored her, and bur-
rowed through the cups on the coffee table. Mrs. Rolla
became exasperated and repeated "Lowell, I said NO!"
Lowell ignored her and picked up a cup. With a resigned
sigh, she filled the cup with water, saying "But do *not* take
it into the doctor's office!" Lowell drank all the water and
carried the cup into the office. Mrs. Rolla heaved another
sigh and sat down in the "patient's chair" next to my desk.
Lowell asked for a toy.

When I gave Lowell permission to play with the toys,
he began pushing a truck around the room, banging it into
our feet. The following interview ensued:

Dr.	Can you tell us about the problems you'd like help with?
Mrs. R.	Just everything with Lowell, like I told the lady on the phone. My neighbor has a hyperactive boy and she says he's just like Lowell, but I didn't want to use her pills until I asked somebody.
Dr.	Good!
Mrs. R.	He just never minds at all. Lowell, stop banging peoples' feet! [Lowell bumped her feet again twice, then roared off. Mrs. R. sighed.]
Dr.	Is that the problem you're talking about?
Mrs. R.	What?
Dr.	Well, just now you asked Lowell to stop, and he continued for a little bit before he stopped.
Mrs. R.	That's it—he never stops.
Dr.	Just now he stopped, but only after he had bumped you a few more times.
Mrs. R.	He never minds unless. . . . Well, sometimes I *do* lose my temper and hit him.
Dr.	How does he respond to that?

Mrs. R.   I don't think it really helps. I don't know what to do [she bursts into tears].

Dr.   How long have things been difficult with Lowell?

Mrs. R   [thinking a moment]. Well, in fact they've never been really good, I mean I've never felt like I was the right mother for him.

Dr.   What was he like as a baby?

Mrs. R.   Do you want the truth? [She glances toward Lowell and pauses.] A great big pain in the ass [weeping]. I don't want to talk about that any more right now with him in the room.

Dr.   OK. Lowell, how would it be if your Mommy waited in the waiting room for a bit while you and I talk?

Lowell.   NO! [He runs to his mother.]

Mrs. R.   Now, Lowell, I'll just be *right* outside the door, and I'll just be gone for a *minute*. I'll just go outside and smoke a cigarette and be right back, and you talk to the doctor. [She leaves, and the clinician places himself between Lowell and the door.]

Lowell.   I WANT MY MOMMY! [Lowell throws a block, which hits the door. He then sits on the floor and plays noisily with the truck. The clinician also sits on the floor. After about five minutes, Lowell rolls the truck toward the clinician, pretending that he doesn't want the clinician to see it. The clinician returns it and this becomes a game.] Here, this is logs [puts blocks on the truck].

Dr.   Lowell, do you like to draw?

Lowell.   No.

Dr.	If I asked you to draw, would you?
Lowell.	No.
Dr.	What if I said you *had* to?
Lowell.	I wouldn't.
Dr.	But what if I insisted?
Lowell.	I'd get MAD!
Dr.	How mad?
Lowell.	Really mad!
Dr.	Could you draw a picture of a boy as mad as that—because somebody made him do something he didn't want to do?
Lowell.	YES! This is the stupid doctor being run over by a truck, and this is the boy who's mad driving it.
Dr.	A very nice drawing! Thanks very much.
Lowell.	Can I take it home?
Dr.	May I keep it here?
Lowell.	OK. Can I play with the house?
Dr.	Sure.
Lowell	[arranging the house and dolls]. Here's this stupid ugly kid—here [he throws the boy doll across the room]! That's you! [He laughs long and hard, rolling about on the floor.] Try to get him in the house!
Dr.	[holding the doll]. Can I come in?
Lowell	[speaking for the assembled family]. NO! Go away and don't bother us any more!
Dr.	I want to come in!
Lowell.	NO! GO AWAY!
Dr.	I'm going to cry.

Lowell.   IF YOU DO . . . !

Dr.   Boo-hoo, they threw me out and won't let me in.

Lowell.   SHUT UP!

Dr.   [Pretending to cry]. They. . . .

Lowell.   I SAID SHUT UP! [Lowell grabs the doll and threatens it with his fist, then beats it on the floor.]

Lowell's subsequent play revolved again and again around the themes of isolation and aggression.

During a subsequent visit, we sought information about the family tree and Lowell's developmental history and temperament.

Dr.   How are things with Lowell?

Mrs. R.   The same: no worse, no better.

Dr.   When you were here the last time, you didn't want to say some things in Lowell's presence.

Mrs. R.   Well, I felt so bad when I said he was . . . you know, when I wasn't nice about him. I've tried so hard to love him (she cried again).

Dr.   What was your life like when he was born?

Mrs. R.   Well, pretty crummy. His dad and me had just split up, and I didn't know I was pregnant. I was living with my folks, and I wanted to go back to school. And I did, and Mom took care of Lowell while I went to beautician's school.

Dr.   Have you seen him since?

Mrs. R.   No. Thank god, the . . . son of a bitch.

Dr.   What was he like?

Mrs. R.   You've seen Lowell. That's what he was like—the spittin' image. Sometimes I just see him in

Lowell, in his eyes—when he's so mean, like that. (Further exploration of this important area indicated a clear link between Mrs. R's anger toward her first husband and her difficulties with Lowell, who resembled his father temperamentally and in appearance.)

Dr.	What was Lowell like when he was a baby?
Mrs. R.	Well, like I said, he was just a pain in the ass.
Dr.	What do you mean, in particular?
Mrs. R.	Everything. He wouldn't do nothing right (weeping). I shouldn't blame it on him; I know it's my fault.
Dr.	What do you mean?
Mrs. R.	Well, nothing ever went right. And my sisters, they never had no trouble with their babies, so I know it's just me. But it's hard not to blame it onto him (weeping again).
Dr.	Let me ask some specific things about what Lowell was like as a baby. First, did he move around a lot? [Activity level.]
Mrs. R.	Did Lowell ever stop moving? Did you see him here? You may not believe this, but when I was seven months pregnant, I was embarrassed to go anywhere in public because my dress jumped all the time from him kicking me.
Dr.	At night did he move around a lot?
Mrs. R.	He wore out a crib, just wiggling. Really, he loosened the joints up in it! I couldn't cover him with a blanket; I had to use sleepers. Now, my other one, my Freddie, he just pretty much lay still where you put him at night, and you could just use a blanket over him. But Lowell, he just was *never* still, even at night.

Dr.   Does it take much to set Lowell off? I mean, is he a hair-trigger kid, or does it take a lot to get a reaction out of him? [Reaction threshold.]

Mrs. R.   Well, hair-trigger is a good word for it.

Dr.   And Freddie?

Mrs. R.   He's not nearly so touchy. He reacts to things, but he seems like he's got a longer fuse than Lowell. He's more normal that way. I mean, if you'd kick him he'd yell, but he's not just always ready to explode, like Lowell.

Dr.   When Lowell responds to something, does he tend to respond with a lot of energy? If he laughs, does he laugh really hard, and if he cries, does he cry hard? [Intensity of Reaction.]

Mrs. R.   Well, I'd say so.

Dr.   So, is it like there aren't many shades of gray with him? He tends to be either on or off?

Mrs. R.   I guess so.

Dr.   Was that true when he was a baby too?

Mrs. R.   I guess so.

Dr.   When he was a baby, was it easy to follow a schedule with him with respect to eating and sleeping and so on? [Rhythmicity.]

Mrs. R.   No, it never was. And that was one of the worst things. I guess that was when I started to hate him [weeps]. All my sisters' kids and Freddie, they just seem to get along, but Lowell just seemed like he was fighting me all the time. He never wanted to eat when it was time to eat, and he never wanted to sleep when it was time to sleep. And of course my mother and sisters and everybody was always telling me: "You can't let him get away with that." And I tried.

I just fought him all the time. I got so tired. He'd nap when I wanted to feed him and yell for food when I was asleep. And all the time, my mother saying "You have to make him mind." I guess she was right because with Freddie I never had that trouble.

Dr.   How does he handle changes? For example, when he was a baby, and you fed him a new food that he hadn't had before, what did he do? [Adaptability.]

Mrs. R.   He was a really messy eater. I always had to clean up after him.

Dr.   Did he raise a fuss if you fed him something he hadn't had before?

Mrs. R.   Oh, probably.

Dr.   How did he act when you gave him a bath for the first time?

Mrs. R.   Oh, I don't know. Is it OK if I smoke in here?

Dr.   Sure. What was his mood like? Was he a happy baby or a crabby baby? [Mood.]

Mrs. R.   He was always crabby—well, usually. I wouldn't say he was happy much of the time. Now my Freddie, he's just the exact opposite. He's always cheerful. And the same with all my sisters' kids—I mean it's fun to be around them —but Lowell is pretty sour, most of the time.

So far we have established that the mother's memory of her experience with Lowell indicates the following temperamental traits: high activity level, low response threshold, low degree of rhythmicity, high intensity of reaction, and negative mood. We are not clear about his adaptability. We might investigate his attention span and persistence, approach/withdrawal, and distractibility.

Dr.   Was it easy for him to play alone for a long time in his crib? [Attention span/persistence.]

Mrs. R.   Well, I don't know. I guess so.

Dr.   When he gets interested in something, does he tend to stick with it for a while?

Mrs. R.   Well, sometimes—like the Saturday morning cartoons, for example.

Dr.   How long does he watch them?

Mrs. R.   As long as they're on.

Dr.   What if something else is going on?

Mrs. R.   Well, it depends. But if he's really interested, he stays with it for a long time.

Dr.   The last time you were here he played with one truck for 30 minutes or more. Is that typical of him?

Mrs. R.   Well, yes, if he really likes something.

Dr.   If he's been watching the cartoons and then for some reason gets to doing something else, does he tend to go back to the cartoons? [Distractibility.]

Mrs. R.   Well, like I said: if he's really interested in what he's doing.

Dr.   When he was a baby—when he was hungry and crying for his food and you were getting things ready, would he stop crying if you held him or rocked him?

Mrs. R.   No, I don't think so. He would probably just keep on crying. Like I said, once he's really into doing something, he tends to keep on doing it, just like with that toy truck the other day.

Dr.   When he was a toddler and he'd get into a tantrum about something, could you stop the tantrum by distracting him? For example, if you picked up a toy for him to play with, would he stop crying?

Mrs. R.   No, he wouldn't, that's for sure. He'd just keep it up and keep it up. That's when I'd just get really mad sometimes and hit him, but that didn't seem to do any good either.

Dr.   How does he handle a strange situation? Does he charge into it or does he tend to hang back? [Approach/withdrawal.]

Mrs. R.   Well, I guess in most places he just charges.

Dr.   The last time you were here, he came into the office ahead of you. Is that typical of him?

Mrs. R.   Yes, I guess it is.

Dr.   Was it easy to start new foods with him when he was a baby?

Mrs. R.   Yes, that never was a problem, and I remember one of my sister's kids would spit out new food and she had to mix a new food with another one that he already liked. But Lowell was never like that.

Dr.   It really sounds like you've had quite a hard time with Lowell.

Mrs. R.   That's why I'm here. I hope you can help us. I've about had it. And if he beats up on his brother again, I'm likely to cream him.

Dr.   Do you think you might injure him, really?

Mrs. R.   No, not really. But to tell you the truth [weeping], there are times I'd sure like to.

Dr.   It seems Freddie has been a lot easier.

Mrs. R.   Oh, after Lowell he was just a dream. He was really easy, no troubles at all. I found myself

wishing I didn't have Lowell around so that I
could enjoy him.

We now have a fairly clear idea that Lowell fits the
pattern of the difficult child. To be sure, the data cannot be
called rigorously reliable, but they do give us some information about how Mrs. R. recalls Lowell to have been and
how she experiences him now. His high activity level, tendency to handle novelty by approach, high degree of persistence, long attention span, and low distractibility are
supported by our observations in the office. In this kind of
interview it is often difficult to differentiate between attention span and persistence and the closely related traits involving response threshold, distractibility, and intensity of
reaction. For our purposes, however, the distinction is
probably not critical; clearly, Lowell's temperament has
been part of the challenge that his mother and he have
experienced. Furthermore, Mrs. R. perceives Freddie's
temperament as being much easier than Lowell's. With this
general idea about Lowell's temperament, we are in a
stronger position to obtain his developmental history.

We have already established that Stage I of Lowell's
development (basic trust versus basic mistrust) was dis-
rupted by his lack of rhythmicity; that Stage II (autonomy
versus shame and doubt) was made more difficult because
he was not easily distracted, had a long attention span and
persistence; and that his high activity level, intense reactions, and negative mood adversely affected both stages.

Dr.   Can we back up a bit? I'd like to know more
           about what your life was like when you met
           Lowell's father.

Mrs. R.   I came here to learn about Lowell, and I don't
           understand what you're poking into my life for.

Dr.   I understand your raising the question; it's just
           that you're such an important part of Lowell's

	world that it would be useful to learn something about your life too.
Mrs. R.	OK, but I wish we'd get to the part about helping me with him. Can you help us?
Dr.	I hope so. But before trying to make any suggestions about something as important as your relationship with your son, I want to make sure I understand what's happening.
Mrs. R.	OK, OK. What do you want to know?
Dr.	Well, I'd like to start with what your life was like when you met Lowell's father.
Mrs. R.	Well, it seems like about a million-and-a-half years ago. We were in high school and started dating, and then I got pregnant, and I wanted to get an abortion because I thought maybe I wanted to go to beauty school, and I didn't want a baby right then. But my parents. . . . Well, it was different then and so I quit high school and we had a great big, white, lovely wedding and all that, and we were miserable and hated it. But my mother does tend to run things, so we thought that was just simpler. But it was a big stupid mistake. And then, to top it all off, I lost the baby right after [weeps again]. But we decided, you know, to make the best of a bad deal. But that's all it ever was—a bad deal. Then, when I found out I was pregnant with Lowell, we had already split up, actually. We got divorced later.
Dr.	How was your health?
Mrs. R.	While I was pregnant? OK, I guess. I mostly felt OK. I had a little bleeding during the second month, but then I was OK.
Dr.	Do you remember the delivery?

Mrs. R.   Oh, sure. The doctor gave me a shot in my back, so I was awake and I saw him right away —in fact, I watched him get born.

Dr.   How did he look?

Mrs. R.   Oh, it was really terrific! I was real excited.

Dr.   Did he cry right away?

Mrs. R.   I think so.

Dr.   What was his color like?

Mrs. R.   Just average baby color, I guess.

Dr.   He was pink?

Mrs. R.   I guess so.

Dr.   Did he wiggle and move right away?

Mrs. R.   Yes, I remember him wiggling and kicking on that little table.

Dr.   Did the doctor seem worried about him?

Mrs. R.   No. And as a matter of fact, he right away started sewing me up again and all that.

Dr.   How soon did you get to hold him?

Mrs. R.   Well, for a minute right away, and then for the first time I fed him, later on.

Dr.   What was feeding him like?

Mrs. R.   I hope I never see that nurse again.

Dr.   What?

Mrs. R.   You just reminded me of that nurse who brought him in. I tried to feed him, and he just wouldn't take the bottle and eat, and the other girl there in the room—I went to high school with her, and she had her baby the same day and she was breast feeding, and the baby just ate fine. Lowell just fussed and spit and carried on, and the nurse said he knew I should be breast-feeding him [she weeps]. And later it was like that with my sisters, because their babies did just fine and ate right from the first and all that. Lowell always made it a hassle.

Dr.   From the *very* first?

Mrs. R.   Yes, I guess so.

Dr.   How long were the two of you in the hospital?

Mrs. R.   Only a few days.

Dr.   Was Lowell OK?

Mrs. R.   As far as they were concerned, yeah. But he and I just weren't hitting it off.

Dr.   What was that like?

Mrs. R.   Well, it was just a constant hassle, like I said. He was screaming for food when I wanted to sleep, and I was trying to feed him when he wanted to sleep, and his dad and I were hassling, and then we split up for good, and then I went to live with my folks again, with Lowell.

Dr.   Did Lowell's father help you with him?

Mrs. R.   Not really. We weren't living together much then.

Dr.   How did he handle the situation when you had difficulties with Lowell?

Mrs. R.   Well, he just made it all a lot worse. He just said: "What's the matter with you? Why can't you take care of your baby?" That could be a part of why we split up, I guess. We just hassled about Lowell all the more. So I thought I'd get away from it all and go back to my folks, but it wasn't all that much different.

Dr.   How so?

Mrs. R.	Well, my folks and sisters just kept telling me to be more patient with him and pointing out that the *other* kids did OK but Lowell and I kept hassling. I guess I got pretty depressed.
Dr.	I can see why.
Mrs. R.	What did I do wrong?
Dr.	Maybe you expected too much of yourself.
Mrs. R.	I just wanted to be a good mother.
Dr.	Lowell would have been a challenge for anyone, and you tackled a tough job without much support, if any. It's no wonder you had a tough time.
Mrs. R.	What do you mean?
Dr.	Well, just by the draw of the cards, you happened to wind up with a child who was a challenge, just because of his temperament.
Mrs. R.	I don't get it.
Dr.	Kids are different, and the way they behave is just as different as the way they look.
Mrs. R.	Yeah, but we had trouble right away, so it had to be me.
Dr.	No, not altogether. Lowell was a challenging boy from the moment he was born. Anyone would have had more difficulty with him than with most other children.
Mrs. R.	You're just blaming it all on him now.
Dr.	No. It's just that the basic, unvarnished Lowell is a real handful. No fault of his or anyone else's.
Mrs. R.	Just one of those things?
Dr.	Just one of those things.

Mrs. R   [silent for a moment]. Far out! You mean my mother and sisters were wrong? That it wasn't just a matter of being more patient?

Dr.   It looks that way.

Mrs. R.   God, I wish I had known!

Dr.   I'd like to know more about his first year. Did he gain weight OK?

Mrs. R.   Yeah, the doctor said he was all right and growing up like he should. He wasn't sickly or anything.

Dr.   When did he first walk?

Mrs. R.   Well, I kept a baby book, and he did everything about when he was supposed to. He was just a year when he first walked. [Lowell's motor development has been normal.]

Dr.   What was it like for you when Lowell started moving around on his own? [Stage II.]

Mrs. R.   Things just kept getting worse. I just can't stop him from doing things, and my mother and sisters keep telling me that I have to be firm and I can't let him get away with anything, but I just can't seem to do it. . . .

Dr.   How did toilet training go?

Mrs. R.   Well, I was determined he wasn't going to get the best of me on *that* issue, and we just battled and battled. I'd set him on the pot and he'd just sit there, and then finally I'd get tired of the whole situation and feel sorry for him and take him off, and then he'd go in his pants. Sometimes I'd lose my temper and whale him a good one, and then I'd feel guilty.

Dr.   Is he toilet trained now?

Mrs. R. Well, he just sort of trained himself all of a sudden, when he was 3½, because he watched a little boy next door and he wanted to be like him [weeps]. That's what's so hard. He makes things hard for me just on *purpose.* Honest to God, I think he lies awake nights trying to figure out ways to bug me.

Dr. Has he had friends?

Mrs. R. Well, that's a sad thing. I think he never has really had a friend for very long. He always breaks their toys or beats them up, and he just doesn't seem to know how to get along with other kids. The kids in the neighborhood are starting to gang up on him, and his little brother is afraid of him.

Dr. Has he ever had a friend for more than six months?

Mrs. R. No, he hasn't.

Dr. Does he do things outside the house?

Mrs. R. No, he really doesn't. He just likes to stay in, and he hangs on me all the time to where I just can't stand it, but there's nothing else he wants to do. The kids don't want to play with him, and he just busts up their toys.

Dr. How did he handle the situation when his half-brother was born?

Mrs. R. Well, he didn't. He just got crabbier and crabbier. He's never liked Freddie, and I've been afraid he was going to really hurt him.

Dr. Has Lowell ever seen his real father?

Mrs. R. No. He came by once and wanted to see Lowell, but my husband got mad because he figured he was trying to see me and he run him off. Lowell was about four then, and he threw a real humdinger about that. He just couldn't understand. Of course, we tell him all the time that we love him just as much as the other boy and so on.

Dr.   Does your husband intend to adopt Lowell?

Mrs. R.   I guess he could, and he says he might, but he says it's not fair to Lowell. To tell the truth, I think he wants to see Lowell straightened out a little before he gives him his name. But he tells Lowell that just because the other boy has Daddy's name and he doesn't, that don't make no difference. I think he really wants to love Lowell, but Lowell just does everything he can to make it hard for him.

Dr.   Do they spend any time together?

Mrs. R.   They used to before Freddie was born, but now, to tell the truth, I think my husband prefers Freddie a little. In fact, we fight about that, but I swear I fear for Lowell if he beats up on Freddie one more time when his dad is around.

Dr.   I'd like to know more about your own family. Do your relatives live in town?

Mrs. R.   Oh, yeah. The whole bunch.

Dr.   Do you see them often?

Mrs. R.   Not really. I don't know what you'd call often. I guess we see my folks about once a week, when we go over there or they come to our place for dinner, but I don't see them too much otherwise—I see my sisters during the week. But I've kind of stopped seeing them so much.

Dr.   Why?

Mrs. R.   Because of Lowell. I'm really tired of hearing

them brag about how sweet their kids are—and they are, really—when I get nothing but flak about Lowell and how he is and how I should do this or that about it. But I've noticed that none of them wants to baby-sit him.

Dr.   Is there any one person in your family who has a big share of the say in most things?

Mrs. R.   Well, I don't know. I guess Mom, in a way. She has a way of predicting things, and you know, she's right a lot of the time. We all joke about that.

Dr.   What happens when someone wants to do something other than what she wants?

Mrs. R.   Well, people just don't. But she's awfully good hearted, and she doesn't meddle. She used to; she'd come over without calling first, just after we got married and we lived nearby. But Ed got mad about that, and first he and I had some fights about it, and I said "After all, she's my mother," and then I saw it more his way. But to tell the truth, I couldn't stand to tell her, so finally Ed did, and she was pretty hurt. But I guess it's worked out OK, although she's always teasing Ed, in her way, you know?

Dr.   About what?

Mrs. R.   Well, just about little things. It don't amount to nothing, but it danders him up some.

Dr.   Is there anyone in your family who doesn't live in the area?

Mrs. R.   I have a brother; he's 27 and he's pretty well out of touch with us. He joined the army right out of high school, and he came back just long enough to get his stuff and then he left right away and married a girl and they have a family.

Dr.	How often do you hear from them?
Mrs. R.	Not very often. He sends us all a Christmas card.
Dr.	How is he doing? [What are the consequences of deviating from family norms?]
Mrs. R.	Not very good. The girl he married seems to sort of take advantage of him, and I understand he's starting to drink, maybe more than he should.
Dr.	Does anyone else in your family drink a lot? [Does the family play any life games?]
Mrs. R.	Well, my dad did. He used to go on these binges every once in a while and be gone for maybe a week or two, drinking and all.
Dr.	Does he drink now?
Mrs. R.	No. He's sober as a judge.
Dr.	What happened?
Mrs. R.	Well, you won't believe this—you're a psychiatrist, so of course you don't believe in religion —but he got religion, and he's been stone sober ever since, and he goes to church twice a week.
Dr.	When did that happen?
Mrs. R.	He had his conversion at a revival about—let's see, it was when I was in high school.
Dr.	Did things change in your family around that time?
Mrs. R.	Well, I don't know. That was about the time Ed and I met, and it wasn't too long after that that I got pregnant. [Was her pregnancy a replacement for her father's alcoholism?]
Dr.	You mentioned that your mother sometimes

predicts things. Can you give me some examples?

Mrs. R.   Well, let's see. She tends to predict—*predict* is too strong a word. She's just joking really, and we all know that. She used to kid me that I'd get pregnant and have to marry some worthless bum. Which I did, as a matter of fact.

Dr.   What does she say about Lowell?

Mrs. R.   Not much good, I'm sorry to say. But then that's probably pretty much true about all of us, I guess.

Dr.   What does she say about him?

Mrs. R.   She says that sometimes he reminds her of her no-good brother Mel.

Dr.   Tell me about Uncle Mel.

Mrs. R.   Well, I never met him, but I guess he was just the bad actor of the family.

Dr.   How bad?

Mrs. R.   Pretty bad, I guess. He spent some time in jail and stuff like that, and he was married several times and left his wives with kids, and never took care of them, and he used to drink a lot too. In fact, I think Lowell kind of looks like him.

Dr.   Now, what does your mother say when she compares Lowell and Uncle Mel?

Mrs. R.   She's just joking you understand. . . . I want you to understand that she's a very good-hearted person; I mean she wouldn't hurt a flea. Really! But anyway, sometimes she jokes that unless I get him straightened out, he'll turn out just like Uncle Mel [weeps]. I wish she wouldn't say that; it gets me so uptight.

Dr.	What would she do if you said you wished she wouldn't say that?
Mrs. R.	She'd just ignore it unless I made a great big federal case out of it. That's what it would take, a federal case.
Dr.	What would happen then?
Mrs. R.	Well, she's very sensitive, of course, and very easily hurt, and she'd be all bent out of shape if she ever felt that I thought she was being unkind or anything. I just couldn't bear to hurt her like that. None of us could. She's always helped us when we were in trouble, and she's so good hearted that none of us could ever bear to say anything like that.
Dr.	Well, if you were to tell your mother that you wished she wouldn't say that about Lowell, and you made a point of it to the extent that she heard what you had to say, what would be the final result after time had passed and the dust had settled?
Mrs. R.	I don't know. I don't think it would change anything.
Dr.	Has anyone ever confronted your mother about anything like that?
Mrs. R.	Well, only once that I remember. Dad and Mom had one big fight that I remember, just before Dad went to that revival. I don't know what started it, but he was yelling at her about something. I never heard anybody yell at her before, and my Dad never yelled at anybody.
Dr.	Did things change after that? [Do the family rules permit structural (Type II) changes?]

Mrs. R.   I don't know. That was when Dad went to the revival and got religion and stopped drinking.

Dr.   How did your mother react to that?

Mrs. R.   OK, I guess. She kids him, in her way, that he's still got the devil in him somewhere. What's all this got to do with Lowell? He's at the baby-sitter's tearing everything up. I have a hard time trying to find a baby-sitter who'll take him.

Dr.   You have a very close family, and they live nearby, and you see them weekly or so. So of course that's an important part of Lowell's life.

Mrs. R   But my parents getting in a fight has got nothing to do with Lowell.

Dr.   Maybe it does.

Mrs. R.   You mean you think that just because my parents got in a fight, that's why Lowell is screwed up? You psychiatrists are nuts.

Dr.   I didn't say that there was any simple link between things, but it is important to understand what the world that Lowell lives in is like.

Mrs. R.   OK, OK. When are you going to tell me how to straighten him out?

Dr.   I'll do my best as soon as I feel I can say something useful.

Mrs. R.   I hope that's pretty soon. I've about had it.

Let's consider the information we have gathered so far. The identified patient, Lowell, lives in a household where, at best, one parent welcomes him. He is threatened further by the presence of a sibling who is welcomed by both parents and was an easy baby, whereas Lowell was a difficult one. Mr. Rolla, who is predisposed by his own ordinal position to find Lowell a difficult problem, says he does not want to adopt Lowell "because it would be unfair to Lowell." The social unit clearly includes Lowell's maternal grandparents and aunts. His maternal grandmother exerts a considerable amount of power in the family, and her power is consolidated by her goodness, sensitivity, and ability to avoid ego-dystonic material through a variety of maneuvers. A major crisis occurred in Mrs. Rolla's family of origin just before Lowell's conception, when her father experienced a religious conversion and stopped drinking. The grandmother views Lowell as prone to becoming the next "bad actor" in the family, and the probability that her prediction will come true seems likely because his temperament and appearance clearly predispose him to this risk.

The degree of differentiation in this family is not high, probably falling within Level 2. Although Mrs. Rolla repeatedly assures us that her mother is only joking when she offers predictions and criticisms, it is clear that these comments are effective means of correcting deviations from the reference structure. Therefore, the family is likely to follow her reference structure, regardless of her conscious desires.

We need to know more about Mr. Rolla's family of origin.

Mr. R.	I never see them.
Dr.	Why is that?
Mr. R.	Well, I was treated fairly rough as a kid, and when I was old enough, I right away quit high school and joined the Marines—and I saw that I could cut it, and I figured I didn't have to put up with that crap from my dad.
Dr.	What do you mean?
Mr. R.	He liked to see me fight. He'd pay me to fight, in fact. I wonder now if he didn't pay the other

	kids too. Then, when I got bigger, he'd take me to bars, and always a fight would start and I'd be in the thick of it. I got damn tired of dragging other guys off his back.
Dr.	So you don't see your family much?
Mr. R.	I don't see them at all. I swore I'd never speak to that son of a bitch again. And I haven't.
Dr.	Where do they live?
Mr. R.	Across town.
Dr.	How long since you've seen them?
Mr. R.	Well, I guess two years last Christmas. We made the mistake of going over there Christmas Day, and that was the last.

Mr. Rolla's self-imposed exile from his own family of origin places even more emphasis on the mythology of his wife's family. Furthermore, a person who leaves a family with a violent wrench, as Mr. Rolla did, may well carry with him the patterns he seeks to escape and, tragically, see them emerge in his children. The extreme effort required to establish a reasonable degree of autonomy from his family suggests a fairly low degree of differentiation. Thus there is a pattern of violent behavior in his family of origin and in his wife's son. We are interested in Mr. Rolla's ordinal position in his family:

Dr.	Do you have brothers and sisters?
Mr. R.	No. My folks tried for a long time to have a kid before me I was the only one.

Lowell's height, weight, head circumference, hearing, dentition, and vision are normal. He is well developed and well nourished and shows right-sided dominance of eyes, hands, and feet. His gross and fine motor coordination, speech, and ability to draw and copy are normal for his age.

We observe no abnormality of thought content or thought processes. His drawings and play reflect the themes of isolation and aggression outlined earlier. Clinical observations confirm a history of a difficult temperament characterized by a high level of activity, low threshold to stimuli, and high intensity of reaction. All this data can be used to generate an initial working formulation and plan of treatment. The case can be written up as follows:

Identifying Data

The identified patient, Lowell Rolla, is an Anglo male; age 4 years, 2 months; born November 15, 1969. The family is self-referred; socioeconomic group 3. No previous therapy. Lowell is the oldest of two children; his younger half-sibling is two years old. The living unit includes Lowell, his half-brother, his mother, and her second husband, who has not adopted Lowell.

Clinical Problem

Chief complaints. The major complaints expressed by Lowell's mother and stepfather are "He won't mind." "He just tries to make things hard." "He beats up on his little brother."

Lowell's play presents themes of isolation and aggression.

Duration and evolution of the problem. According to Mrs. Rolla, Lowell was difficult from the beginning. He has become increasingly belligerent and hostile toward his younger brother in recent months. There are no clear-cut exacerbating or relieving environmental circumstances. So far as we know, there are no instances of a good relationship between Lowell and his half-sibling or stepfather. His relationship with his mother has always been strained; she has never enjoyed him.

Temperamental Type

Difficult, with a low response threshold, high activity level, and intense reactions that are clearly evident in his history and in the office.

Developmental History

Identified patient. Lowell has always been in good health. His development has been complicated throughout by his difficult temperament, the stigma of being the son of a "bum" and the result of a premature and unwanted pregnancy, and by the presence of numerous relatives who continually admonish his mother to "correct" him and make him behave like his temperamentally easy cousins. His physical and psychological development has been normal, with the exception of his extremely poor peer relationships.

His parents divorced in his infancy. His mother remarried when he was two, and his step-sibling was born when he was 2½.

Mother. Mrs. Rolla is the third of four daughters. Her father, who reformed after experiencing a religious conversion, was an alcoholic during her childhood. Her mother remains a highly dominant force in her life and has exerted influence in the family through "joking" predictions.

She has always been competitive with her older sisters, feeling that she could never be as good as they were. The family has always lived in the same neighborhood.

Step-father. Lowell's step-father, an only child, has created a strong barrier between himself and his family of origin. He was encouraged to fight other youngsters during boyhood and men during adolescence. Having left his family with much anger and bitterness, he describes his in-laws in glowing terms.

Family Tree

The family tree holds a wealth of information (see Figure 9.1). According to Mrs. Rolla, Lowell is the "spittin' image

of his dad," who is "a son-of-a-bitch." Lowell's development is complicated by a difficult temperament, in contrast
to his half-brother's easy one. On the level of the extended
family, we note that the maternal grandmother, who is
prone to make predictions, wields considerable power in
the family.

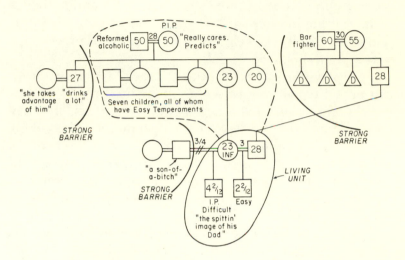

Figure 9.1   The Rolla Family Tree
GENERAL INFORMATION

Degree of Differentiation

The presence of strong barriers and alliances, a clear person in power, alcoholism, and the physical proximity of
family members suggests a fairly low level of differentiation
—probably Level 2.

Four Parameters of Family Function

Anxiety. Mrs. Rolla ranks high in anxiety, Mr. Rolla and the
maternal grandmother seem to rank low. Although Lowell's anxiety level is hard to assess, it is probably not
low.

Capacity to Change. We cannot assess at this point the capacity of family members to change. The repetition of patterns in the family tree, particularly the pattern of rescue (Mr. Rolla rescued his father from fights, and alcoholism is a form of the Game of Rescue in his wife's family) raise serious doubts about the system's ability to change. The relationship between Lowell's mother and grandmother is of special importance in this regard, and careful exploration of Mrs. Rolla's developmental history and current support system might be useful.

Sympton-carrier role. Obviously, Lowell is the symptom carrier. Of equal interest is the possibility that his grandmother and stepbrother are "super clean": that is, they may be considered beyond reproach. His stepfather's loss of his own family of origin, with the resulting oversupport of his wife's family, as well as the overinvestment that we would expect an only child to have in his son, might tend to strengthen this pattern. Lowell's difficult temperament, of course, is an additional influence.

Power. The assessment of power is difficult. The grandmother's predictions about the behavior of other family members indicate that she in fact wields considerable power. The consequences of diverging from the accepted family pattern would apparently be painful for all concerned. Since the sibling who left the family does not seem to be doing well, others will not be encouraged to follow his example.

These preliminary estimates generate the following chart:

Dimension	Low	High
Anxiety	Lowell	Mrs. Rolla
Capacity to change	Mrs. Rolla	
Symptom-carrier role	Grandmother Freddie	Lowell
Power	Mrs. Rolla	Grandmother?

Let us digress into a discussion of this chart; these comments might not be appropriate in a workup. If our estimates are correct, the grandmother is in a highly vulnerable position, especially if the family's degree of differentiation is as low as we have estimated (i.e., if Commoner's rule that everything is connected to everything else in fact applies fairly consistently). These speculations have the following clinical implications:

1. If the family is poorly differentiated, if the grandmother is vulnerable when change occurs, if therapy results in changes in the family, and if the family maintains its balance through the Game of Rescue, then the grandmother may become ill.

2. If change increases the grandmother's anxiety, the family may decide that treatment for Lowell is too expensive and may terminate it.

3. The four-dimensional chart and the family tree indicate that a significant part of the case will involve Mrs. Rolla's ability to assess Lowell's behavior realistically and protect him from the destructive mythology of her second husband and her family of origin. If shifts involve a significant power struggle between Mrs. Rolla and her mother, the result may be extreme turbulence throughout the entire family. Will giving Lowell a fair chance require his mother to grieve the loss of her own family or her second marriage?

4. If Mrs. Rolla and her mother come into conflict, they may move into a dangerous and unstable configuration that will generate anxiety in both, an active power struggle may occur, neither will want to accommodate in any major way, and each will try to scapegoat the other. If this happens, the rule that unstable dyads become triads will probably apply, and a third person will be called on to tip the balance decisively one way or the other. Therefore, Mr. Rolla may be crucial in determining whether Lowell will be allowed to occupy a healthy niche in the family.

5. It might be useful to seek an initial evaluative session with the entire, extended family on the grounds that the entire family is important.

6. The therapist should carefully avoid overidentifying with Lowell and directing inappropriate anger toward Mrs. Rolla or her mother.

Clinical Observations

Identified patient. Lowell is a well-developed, well-nourished, strong-looking four-year-old who is alert, active, and occasionally cooperative. He shows no indication of significant biological disorder. His temperament is characterized by a low threshold to stimuli, high level of activity, and high intensity of reaction. His drawings and play reveal themes of isolation and aggressiveness directed toward others. Interpersonally, he is somewhat negativistic, although not unmanageably so. There is no evidence of mental retardation or thought disorder. His gross and fine motor functions are normal, as are his sensory and sensory-motor functions. His affect is consistent with the themes of isolation and hostility that occur during play.

Other family members. Mrs. Rolla is a tired-looking, seemingly depressed young woman who looks slightly older than her stated age of 23. There is no evidence of mental abnormality, and she relates appropriately to the examiner. Her concern about Lowell, her inability to manage him, and her anxiety seem appropriately focused. Although she seems to perceive her son's difficulties as arising from her failure as a mother, she is able to respond appropriately to an alternative explanation.

Her interactions with Lowell are characterized by agreeing to his demands after a period of denial and thus creating a variable reinforcement pattern.

Mr. Rolla was willing to come to the office for a brief

interview, but he was moderately annoyed when the examiner suggested that he was important and considered the difficulties to lie between Lowell and his wife. Although he verbally expressed interest and concern for Lowell, his nonverbal communication led the examiner to believe that Mr. Rolla's life would improve if Lowell conveniently disappeared.

Mrs. Rolla would not permit us to contact her mother by telephone because her mother might misinterpret our reasons for doing so and cause difficulties within the family.

Formulation

Biological. The identified patient, age four years and five months, is the oldest of two boys. He is in good health, has no medical difficulties, and his temperament is characterized by a high level of activity, low threshold to stimuli, and intense reactions.

Developmental. Lowell was a "shotgun" child; his parents divorced when he was two, with subsequent arrival of a half-brother by his mother's second husband. Progressive scapegoating by members of extended family, with increasing identification with the family "bad guy," Mrs. Rolla's Uncle Mel. The maternal grandmother, the person in power, predicts that the patient will be at high risk for bad behavior. His interactions with his mother have increased her dislike of him while reinforcing, through a variable-ratio schedule, his progressively more demanding behavior. Difficulties occurred in the mother-infant system concerning feeding, and there were subsequent problems with toilet training and other power issues during toddlerhood.

Current situation. The identified patient lives with his mother, half-brother and stepfather. The social unit includes the mother's sisters and the patient's cousins, who are perceived as "good children." His half-brother is a competent, likable, pleasant two-year-old who is welcomed warmly into the nuclear and extended family.

Coping maneuvers. Lowell responds to the stresses of his current environment with what appears to be an exacerbation of his normal behavior. Specifically, he demonstrates negativism, which his mother reinforces, and hostility toward his younger brother. The reversibility of his symptomatic behaviors, including his excessive hostility toward his half-brother and his poor peer relationships, cannot be assessed at this point.

Differential Diagnosis (using GAP Report No. 62)

Healthy responses. The predominant themes of aggression and isolation in Lowell's play and his inappropriate social functioning eliminate this factor as a major consideration.

Reactive disorder. The intensity and severity of Lowell's hostility toward peers and his half-brother suggest a possible reactive disorder. The history, however, indicates that Lowell and his mother have been a marginally functional dyad from his early infancy; Freddie's birth seems to have exacerbated patterns that were already present. Therefore, although the current difficulties could certainly be related in part to Lowell's reaction to his mother's new family, from which he is excluded, this diagnosis does not appear adequate.

Developmental deviations. This category merits consideration because there is evidence of a significant biological contribution (temperament), because Lowell's symptomatic behaviors are beyond the normal range, and because the reversibility of these patterns can be seriously questioned at this time. We might evaluate Lowell in terms of his social, psychosexual, and affective development.

Although his age precludes a firm diagnosis, Lowell may be at risk for psychoneurotic disorder, personality disorder (e.g., oppositional, tension-discharge, or sociosyntonic type), or some other diagnostic consideraton such as hyperactivity.

Target Problems and Intervention Plans

In summary, Lowell Rolla's development has been complicated by complex interactions on all levels (biological, psychological, family, and social). The clinician must carefully assess the relative importance of each and the cost-benefit ratio of reasonable interventions.

Psychosexual Level	Target Problems	Intervention Plans
Biological	Hyperactivity	Further observation; further workup as indicated
Psychological	Agressiveness	Individual therapy may be indicated
	Isolation	Family counseling or therapy may be indicated
Family	Scapegoating Extrusion	Family therapy may be indicated
	Physical hazard to half-sibling	This issue might be explored with the parents.
	Hazard to grandmother's health in case of a shift in family balance	Observe the family closely for signs of impending distress; be prepared for clinical resistance and try to assess the basis for it.
	Mother's variable reinforcement of bad behavior	Individual therapy for the mother might be considered at some point.
	Mother's depression	
	Step-father's difficulty in accepting Lowell	Counseling or therapy with one or both parents might be indicated.
Social	Poor peer relations	This issue may emerge in individual therapy. At some point Lowell may be a candidate for group therapy.

JOHN CROWELL

Our first contact with John Crowell occurred when he was 13 years old. The family requested psychological testing since they were concerned that John might have a "specific learning disability." They had read "some of the more recent literature" about learning disabilities and wanted a comprehensive evaluation of the problem.

John and his parents arrived a few minutes before the appointed hour in an expensive car. They were impeccably, fashionably, and conservatively dressed. In the waiting room, Mr. and Mrs. Crowell sat on the same couch in similar postures, reading books they had brought with them. John sat in a chair about ten feet away, slouching somewhat and staring vacantly at his feet. Over a period of five minutes, no one changed his posture.

Dr.	Hello, are you the Crowell family? [The parents stood and shook hands with the clinician, who introduced himself to all three.]
Mr. C.	Stand up, John. [John stood.]
Dr.	Would you like to come into the office? [At his parent's suggestion, John entered the room first and sat, slouching, in the "patient's chair." His parents seated themselves primly.]
Mr. C.	We understand that this clinic has a university affiliation. Is that correct?
Dr.	Yes.
Mrs. C.	Are you board certified?
Dr.	No.
Mr. C.	Are you board eligible?
Dr.	Yes.
Mrs. C.	To tell the truth, we checked into your creden-

tials before we came. We were sure you
wouldn't mind.

Dr.   I don't mind.

Mr. Crowell, an attorney, holds an important administrative position in a large manufacturing firm. The Cro-
wells are wealthy because of Mr. Crowell's earnings and a
large inheritance; the family lives a secluded, highly respectable life in a secluded, highly respectable neighborhood. John is the third of four children: Alex is the oldest,
the second and fourth are daughters, Judy and Mary.

Dr.   What do you want us to help you with?

Mr. C.   Did you have the opportunity to review the
               material from the other clinics?

Dr.   I have the reports, but I thought it would be
               best if I spoke to you directly first.

Mrs. C.   Well, we're hoping for a thorough evaluation,
               and I'm sure you'll review the material care-
               fully.

Dr.   Certainly.

Mr. C.   The truth is, doctor—and I am certain that I
               may speak confidentially—we are a bit finan-
               cially embarrassed at the moment, having
               found care of John to be quite a burden—
               financially speaking.

John has been evaluated by a number of clinicians and
has been given numerous diagnostic labels. We discover
that he was in therapy for four years, three sessions per
week, with the area's most expensive and prestigious therapist, but there was little or no discernible change.[1] During
John's therapy, his parents saw a social worker once a week.
But we still lack a chief complaint.

Dr.	What do you want us to help you with?
Mrs. C.	John.
Mr. C.	John simply doesn't measure up.

Mr. Crowell, the son of poor immigrants, is enormously proud of being a self-made man. His parents are now dead; he is an only child and has no close relatives. Mrs. Crowell is the youngest child of a wealthy family that is well established in the area.

Dr.	It sounds like your problems with John are fairly global: "He doesn't measure up."
Mr. C.	Well, I'd have to agree. Wouldn't you, dear?
Mrs. C	[nods and begins to cry]. After all we've done . . . and he still won't give us what we want.
Dr.	Can you clarify what you want? Can you help me understand what you've experienced?
John.	They just think I'm going to be like my brother.
Dr.	Tell me about your brother.
John.	Well, he just hangs around the Haight-Ashbury district and smokes pot, and doesn't work or anything.
Mr. C	[visibly enraged]. That's not true! He is in business now, and he is working at it quite steadily.
Mrs. C	[speaking quietly]. Now, dear, we don't really know that. We don't really know *how* it's going. Of course, we do know that he does have a business now.
Dr.	What is he doing?
Mr. C.	He owns and operates a small specialty store.
John.	He doesn't own it, and he doesn't operate it.
Mr. and Mrs. C	[virtually in unison]. John! Be more respectful!

The clinician notes a faint smile on John's face. It fades and John resumes his slouched position and stares at his feet. Clearly, these parents struggle to maintain their composure in every aspect of their lives. It will therefore be difficult to extract key information from this family system. Their discomfort about discussing important material despite years of therapy suggests an inability to change. The close agreement between the two and their tight control over John suggest a low degree of differentiation. The brief but vigorous exchange just observed—like any crisis, however minor—helps to shake some data from this rigid family. The following four-place chart illustrates these exchanges.

Dimension	Low	High
Anxiety	John	
	Parents	
Capacity to change	John	
	Parents	
Symptom-carrier role	Parents	John
Power	John	Parents

Initially, no one seems especially anxious, although the parents' anxiety apparently exceeds John's. The capacity of all three to change seems low. The initial picture presents John as the symptom carrier and his parents as above reproach. The parents' power is greater than John's. We also note that the parents agree at all times.

The brief conflict, however, moves the family abruptly into the following configuration:

	Low	High
Anxiety	John	Parents
Capacity to change	Parents	
	John?	
Symptom-carrier role	John	Parents
	Parents	John
Power		Parents John

John remains calm, at least outwardly, while both parents are anxious. By challenging the predominant mythology, John may be indicating some capacity to change.

Note that it was necessary to subdivide the symptom-carrier columns. John perceives his parents as symptomatic and himself as nonsymptomatic while his parents view things the other way around; thus the crossed configuration in the third column. Although power is usually the most difficult parameter to assess, the parents' discomfort indicates that John is capable of plunging the family into chaos. Predictably, Mr. and Mrs. Crowell successfully engage John in a power struggle to reestablish their own predominance and reduce their anxiety. But it is clear that John, merely by challenging their perception of their older son, can immediately shift the family into a painful configuration that is immediately recognizable as Ping-Pong or Warfare. We could speculate that if the family was able to tolerate this change in configuration for a brief period, it might become healthier. Furthermore, it is clear that there is some buried mythology about John's older brother.

The chronicity of family patterns and the consequences of change are crucial issues. Therefore, we ask the following question:

Dr.   I noticed that there was a brief flare-up just now. Are those common?

Mr. C.   The fact is, doctor, that they're becoming a lot worse. I hope you won't mind if I take a moment to criticize your profession, but I absolutely can't understand how treatment by a most highly recommended and competent man can make our son worse instead of better. Now, we're here to see if John can be straightened out, and if not, I can assure you that the consequences will be serious. Serious!

Has individual therapy helped John grow to the point where he can now challenge his parents? Perhaps his therapy was successful and the current turmoil reflects this.

Dr.   I see. How do you handle it when John challenges you, as he did just now?

John.   They yell and threaten, and if I keep it up long enough, they hit me.

Dr.   Oh?

Mr. C   [visibly embarrassed]. Now, you must understand that John exaggerates more than a little. I'm sure you understand that it's occasionally necessary to discipline the boy. I'm sure you find it necessary to spank your own children, at least occasionally, and of course for good reason.

Mrs. C.   I wish you wouldn't hit him.

This is a new piece of process. Mr. and Mrs. Crowell are disagreeing for the first time; therefore, the following exchange is likely to provide information about their rules of adaptation.

Mr. C   [stiffens visibly].

John.   I kind of wish you wouldn't hit me, Dad.

John's affect, of course, is important. If he were genuinely frightened, the content and affect of his communication would be coherent, and the message would be a fairly simple one. However, he does not sound frightened; he sounds a bit sassy. The therapist observes a faint grin on his face.

Mrs. C.   In fact, you really shouldn't hit him. I've told you so many times. [She begins to wring her hands and bites her lip.]

Mr. C.	I'LL THANK YOU TO BE RESPECTFUL OF ME WHEN WE'RE IN PUBLIC!
Mrs. C.	We're not in public.
John.	Dad, this is an office.
Mr. C.	[to his wife]. TELL HIM TO SHUT UP!
Mrs. C.	Be quiet, John. Your father is upset.
John.	[turning to the clinician]. Be careful. My father is upset.
Mr. C.	I tell you, Doctor, if that boy doesn't start behaving respectfully, I'll. . . .
Mrs. C.	You'll what, dear?
Mr. C.	I'LL THROW HIM OUT!
Mrs. C.	YOU WILL NOT DO ANYTHING OF THE KIND!
Mrs. C.	Doctor, this is *exactly* how we got into the mess with our older boy. His father just kept pushing and pushing and finally threatened to throw him out. And then he did, and we got word that he was just wasting his life, you know, and . . . [she begins to cry].
Mr. C.	He wouldn't have turned into such a lousy no-good if you hadn't coddled him all his life. This is precisely what happens. You will never permit a reasonable amount of discipline. You always intervene.
Mrs. C.	[visibly angry]. Now, I'll just take you up on that. I'm really tired of your beating the kids and saying it's just fine. I just can't tolerate it, and I won't. You can just get used to that, because I absolutely will not tolerate your abusing our children and then throwing them out! You ruined our first son . . . [weeps again].

The family sits glumly for about three minutes. The ticking of the clock is the only sound in the room.

Mr. C.   [calmly]. We came here to discuss John, and I suggest that we continue with that. John's school performance is far from satisfactory, and it's going to be essential—if he's going to be a man in this world—that he learn to care for himself, and it's essential that he get an education. That's why we're here. I hope you can help us.

MRS. C.   Yes, of course. John's education is the central problem.

During this exchange the parents have been engaged in an active struggle. This configuration can be charted as follows:

		Low	*High*
Anxiety			Mr. C
			Mrs. C
Capacity to change		?	
Symptom-carrier role	Mrs. C's view	Mrs. C	Mr. C
	Mrs. C's view	Mr. C	Mrs. C
Power			Mrs. C
			Mr. C

This is the dangerous Warfare configuration: both parents are anxious, they are engaged in an active power struggle, and neither seems willing to make a major concession. There is active disagreement about which parent is the symptom-carrier: each views himself as reasonable and the other as symptomatic; each struggles to avoid being labelled symptomatic. Notice, however, that the family returns to the initial configuration in which John stares at his feet while his parents calmly agree that he is the problem. The scene is restored to its preconflict state, with no discernible change. The key question now is: *As the family went through this brief configurational change, did it learn anything useful? Did the rigidity of roles increase or decrease?* In other words, we want to know whether this struggle is chronic and how the family responds to it.

Dr.   Are these disagreements common?

Mr. C.   Well, only when John becomes thoroughly impossible.

Mrs. C.   Yes, I'd say that's true. John is doing very poorly in school, and we're very concerned about that, of course. And of course that's a source of much tension in the family.

John.   They fight like that sometimes.

Dr.   Do these fights tend to happen more or less the same way? When you argue, do you tend to use pretty much the same maneuvers getting into the fight and back out of it again?

Mr. C.   I never thought about it that way, but. . . . Well, I don't know; I'd have to think about it. But I think I see what you mean.

In a subsequent interview, we obtained information about John's development (See Table 9.1). This information can be summarized as follows:

Identifying Data

John Crowell, 13-year-old male, born August 14, 1960. Third of four children (male, female, male, female); upper-middle class and upwardly mobile family. Family requested psychological testing after patient had three years of intensive therapy with Dr. Meldon. No apparent major life changes have occurred recently.

Table 9.1 John Crowell's Developmental History

Psychosexual Stage	Biological Development	Psychological Development	Family Status	Social Development
Prenatal	Normal pregnancy and delivery	Desired pregnancy	Stable marriage. Son 12, daughter 7. Father very busy; building career rapidly; he is the rising star of the firm. High expectations for a successful son.	
I. Infancy	Clearly slow-to-warmup temperament. Gained weight slowly	"He never cried. He was always very passive." No response to "peek-a-boo"		Questionable history that he enjoyed "peek-a-boo" game at eight months.
II. Toddlerhood	Generally in good health. No hospitalizations, operations, accidents, injuries, allergies or serious illness of any kind.	No history of power struggles. No descernible response to birth of sister.	Younger sister born when I.P. was three years old.	Played alone and quietly in nursery school.
III. Preschool		"Quiet, withdrawn. He would stand at bedroom door and stare."	The pattern of brief and vigorous parental arguments became more pronounced as difficulties developed concerning Alex	Did not make friends. Seemed confused by other childrens' approaches to him.
IV. Grade School		Psychological testing, sought by parents due to school failure, indicated normal I.Q.		
V. Adolescence	Normal physical-neurological exam.	Increasingly withdrawn. No evidence that he has the ability to establish an identity.		No history of any significant friendships.

Clinical Problem

Chief complaints. Parents: "He doesn't work in school. He doesn't measure up." John has no chief complaint.
Duration and evolution of the problem. Apparently, John's passivity and his parents' dissatisfaction with him are virtually lifelong. No intervention of any kind, including private tutoring and many hours of psychotherapy, have made any discernible difference in John's behavior.

Temperamental Type

Although the parents are not clear about most of John's temperamental traits; the overall pattern is one of a child who is slow to warm up (see Table 9.2).

Table 9.2   Evaluation of John Crowell's Temperamental Type

Trait	Described by Parents		Currently Observed By:
	Infancy	*Childhood*	
Activity Level	Low		not high
Adaptability	?		
Rhythmicity	High		
Mood	?		?
Approach/withdrawal	Withdrawal		
Intensity of reaction	Low		moderate or low
Threshold	?	?	?
Persistence attention span	?		
Distractibility	?		

Developmental History

Identified patient. John has no friends and is not deeply involved in any activity. He has not had any serious illnesses, accidents, or injuries. His developmental course has been normal; but his height and weight have always been below normal.

Other family members. John's older brother, Alex, apparently had a similar life history. He now lives in a large city and seems to be functioning marginally, supported by his parents. John's sisters are asymptomatic.

Mr. Crowell, an only child of poor parents, is a self-made, successful lawyer-businessman. Mrs. Crowell is the oldest of three daughers of a wealthy and prestigious family.

Family Tree

Mr. and Mrs. Crowell live isolated lives. John is vulnerable as the second son of an upwardly mobile father whose oldest son is dysfunctional and of a mother who, as the eldest of three sisters, is likely to prefer her daughters. Mrs. Crowell avoids her family of origin. The Crowell's oldest daughter married at age 18, lives in another state, and actively avoids her family of origin when possible. (See the family tree, Figure 9.2)

Degree of Differentiation

Family members typically remain closely tied to a family of origin or manage to escape by fairly extreme means: e.g., Mrs. Crowell and Judy. Alex's inability to establish an independent source of income has resulted in financial dependence on his family under the guise of managing a business. Clinically, we have observed that Mr. and Mrs. Crowell agree closely on all matters, alternating with brief but vigorous arguments. These observations suggest that the family's level of differentiation is probably not above Level 2.

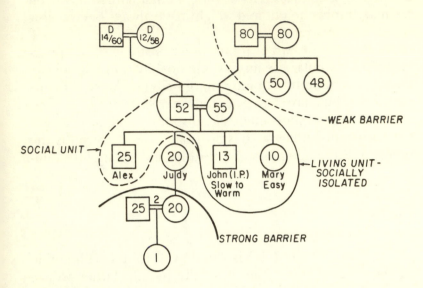

Figure 9.2 The Crowell Family Tree

Four Parameters of Family Function

In general, the family members hold clear and predictable configurations. John is L?HL; his parents are ?LLH. However, these configurations can change rapidly. During an active power struggle, both parents are HL?H (the Ping-pong or Warfare configuration) while John becomes L?LH in his own eyes and L?HH in his parents' eyes.

These patterns seem both extreme and chronic. The shifts in configurations occur abruptly, and one complete rotation from the initial configuration to the Warfare configuration and back again does not seem to result in useful learning.

Clinical Observations

John is a passively cooperative, pleasant, well-dressed young man. He is well-oriented and alert, with no evidence of a thought disorder. Although he seems to lack initiative and intelligence, he occasionally exhibits a remarkable degree of observational ability, initiative, and interpersonal skill—for example, when commenting on his brother.

John's parents are well controlled and well protected in interpersonal interactions, except during disagreements over Alex. They have a penetrating interest in the clinician and seem both respectful and distant. They are obviously angry at John. Their affect is well controlled and humorless.

Formulation

Biological. This 13-year-old boy, the third of four children (male, female, male, female) is temperamentally slow to warm up. His intelligence is average according to previous testing, and his health has been good: twentieth percentile in terms of height and weight. Physical and neurological examinations have been normal.

Developmental. John has been passive since infancy. His physical development has been normal. He has always been quiet and withdrawn interpersonally: e.g., he did not respond to the peek-a-boo game at age eight months and has had no lasting friendships. His school performance has been poor academically, but he presents no disciplinary difficulties.

Current situation. John is now the oldest child living at home. His school performance is especially embarrassing to his parents because of Alex's hippy life-style. John has no friends and his parents do not like him. Despite their outward appearance of concern and tranquility, Mr. and Mrs. Crowell can be thrown into intense conflict if their pain and guilt about Alex is deftly manipulated. John has demonstrated a remarkable ability to do precisely that, and it may serve to deflect his parents' attention from his school failure. Yet John's age and the failure of previous therapy have fanned the flames of the parents' frustration.

Coping Maneuvers. In contrast to his customary lack-luster style, John demonstrates remarkable interpersonal skills, initiative, and timing when disrupting his parents. He apparently has not resorted to any extreme coping maneuvers.

Differential Diagnosis (using GAP Report No. 62)

Healthy responses. John's poor academic and social performance and minimally variable affect rule out healthy responses as a major possibility.

Reactive disorder. Although John's poor academic performance, despite an adequate intelligence, and his poor functioning with peers may be pathological in degree, their occurrence as responses is at best problematic. In any case, the reversibility of these patterns is open to serious question.

Developmental deviations. The chronicity and severity of John's difficulties raises the distinct possibility of a developmental deviation. We might consider the following specific dimension: cognitive functioning, social development, and affective development, particularly chronic depression. Deviation in other areas can by no means be excluded.

Psychoneurotic disorders. John's poor academic performance means that intrapsychic conflict cannot be ruled out at this point. Additional evidence may emerge during individual sessions or testing. Dr. Meldon, who worked with John for several years, may offer a useful opinion.

Personality disorders. John may have incorporated into his personality some maladaptive coping maneuvers, which are now relatively fixed.[1] We might want to investigate the following disorders: overly dependent personality, oppositional personality, overly inhibited personality, isolated personality, and mistrustful personality. Psychotic and psychophysiologic disorders, brain syndromes, and mental retardation do not apply in John's case.

Target Problems and Intervention Plans

Psychosexual Stage	Target Problems	Intervention plans
Biological	Slow-to-warm temperament.	Consider the role of temperament during development. Consider discussion of this factor in an interpretative session with parents.
Psychological	Depression? Personality disorder?	Evaluation of prior records; after obtaining the parents' permission, contact previous therapists about the following: Is John capable of developing his own chief complaint or goals for therapy? Is he capable of a working alliance?
	Significant intrapsychic conflict?	Can he make constructive use of counseling or therapy? Why was his therapy terminated?[1]
Family	Parental conflict, and John's exploitation of it.	Further exploration of this process may be indicated. Proceed, with a maximum amount of attention to the working alliance with the parents, while not "doing to" John. Carefully explore the implications of the initial request and the possibilities of changing the request. (Note: the parents' requested *testing* for John. Are they interested in exploring other areas? Are we willing to do the testing?)
Social	No friends.	Explore history in detail. Has John *ever* had a friend? For how long? Has he ever invested significant interest and energy in a pet? Would John be a candidate for group therapy? When?

Perhaps this chapter should have been titled "Out of the Ivory Tower and into the Streets" for I am certain that other clinicians would have done things differently at many points in these two cases. However, my purpose was not to illustrate a best way but to illustrate the use of clinical tools discussed in earlier chapters. I hope that the problem-plan lists follow logically from the material obtained during interviews with these families.

NOTES

1. Therapy might have been terminated after a realistic assessment that it was having little or no impact on John's symptoms. On the other hand, the parents may have terminated the treatment if John's self-confidence and interpersonal skills improved to a degree that enabled him to exploit the latent discord between his parents. The implications of these divergent possibilities for future work with John and his family are obvious.
2. In general, I assume that any nonpsychotic behavior is or has been adaptive in some context. As used here, the term maladaptive assumes that there may be behaviors which, although adaptive in some situations, are maladaptive in the majority of randomly selected environments.

EPILOGUE

I write this conclusion from a special perspective. More than three years have passed since I first wrote out an outline to use when organizing a child-family workup. Little did I imagine the project that would emerge from that mustard seed. Now, having had the opportunity to work out many of the points raised in this book in some detail in a clinical setting, I am in a better position to think in general terms about how to apply this material. If I saw this manuscript for the first time today, how would I react? What would I do with it?

Like any specialized structure, a clinical style has a lengthy and complex developmental history. Like a personality, it develops in a specific social context, and its configuration reflects adaptation to that context. Therefore, a set of clinical tools designed for use in one clinic may be inappropriate when used in another. What selection biases influence the patient population that comes in? At the outset, major constraints are placed on the kinds of data-gathering tools and interventions that are possible. Ivory-tower thoroughness is wasteful and inefficient. Because clinical teaching is probably responsible for only a small portion of overall clinical expertise, the student must sort out the difficult problem of cost-benefit ratio in a different arena. Therapeutic techniques (both psychodynamic and behavioral) are almost always developed using highly specialized populations such as college students who come to a student health clinic or highly motivated upper middle-class folk. Consequently, transferring these techniques from one clinical setting to another can be frustrating and even dangerous. The same is true of evaluation. A lengthy questionnaire concerning a child's development may be invaluable in one clinic and offensive to parents in another.

This book is of necessity culture-bound because it is written by a white, Anglo-Saxon Protestant male. Clinical tools, like plants must be transplanted carefully into a new environment for the sake of both. Therefore, this book must conclude with the following challenge: you must compose your own evaluative outline, clinical tools, questionnaires, and interventions.

Which principles and practices presented in this book are most general? Let me reexamine a few of them with an eye to this issue.

The slippery but central concept of development must have wide applicability on the level of the family and its rules as well as on the individual level. Translating the concept to clinical use takes many forms. A corollary concept, developmental *lines*, facilitates the translation. For example, biological, cognitive, psychosexual, and social functions can be assessed somewhat independently. It takes years of experience to develop clinical expertise; the printed page can only facilitate this development. Similarly, the distinction between developmental *lag* (development that is on the right track, but slow) and developmental *deviation* (off the track) is useful when translating the concept of development into clinical use. The issue of reversibility then becomes central. Thus, although development is not as crisply defined as it could be, it is possible to look at a variety of functions and seek to differentiate between lag and deviation as well as estimate the reversibility of abnormality regardless of clinical context. The extent to which these issues should be pursued must be a matter of clinical judgment.

Every person develops and lives in a social context. The family tree is one clinical approach to gathering the relevant data. Of all the tools described in this book, the family tree has been the "sleeper." I had no idea that it would become a central method of collecting and organizing data. Not only is it easy to teach, use, and learn, but it is benign from the data-gathering standpoint, yet clinically powerful. The transition from the chief complaint and history of the problem to questions about the extended family can be made easily. Early recognition of the multiproblem family is especially valuable because realistic expectations are essential in these cases. Here the clinician's cultural bias is clearest. In terms of sociocultural environment, the clinician may have more in common with a person from another country and culture than with someone from the same town. Similarities in dress and speech can blind us to the presence of a crucial boundary in terms of family rules.

Complementary to the family tree is the concept of differentiation, which appears to be completely culture free. Although my biases in favor of its direct application as a clinical tool are made clear elsewhere, others have been less than eager to implement it. The selection biases of a particular setting may present the clinician with such a narrow range of the entire spectrum that attempts to assess the degree of differentiation in each case may be uselessly redundant. In any case, the concept of differentiation may be a useful back-up tool. If a clinician is having difficulties with a case, he would be wise to reconsider the level of differentiation of the identified patient and family. How much work will be necessary for them to move a given behavioral distance? If we underestimate the amount of work by overestimating the level of differentiation, we are likely to become angry and resentful, inferring unfairly that the patient and family are not motivated or are not working.

The astute have already noted some isomorphism between degree of differentiation and psychosexual level. That is, a family described as poorly differentiated and operating at Level 1 will contain individuals who are primarily involved with issues of basic trust. Similarly, individuals in families at level 2 are likely to be dealing with issues of autonomy versus shame and doubt. This similarity of form between the psychosexual stages of individual development described by Freud and Erikson and the five levels of differentiation proposed by Hoover and Franz (1972) and used in this book as opposed to the four levels proposed by Bowen (1966), may be clinically convenient. It also *may* be theoretically sound, but we must not allow clinically convenient shorthand to short-circuit our more critical thought processes.

In any case, an awareness of the "stickiness" of the social field is essential. In a homogeneous patient population, this may be done only once and then assumed. In some clinical settings it may be an essential part of each evaluation.

The sociocultural bias of this book is most clearly illustrated by the brevity of the discussion about the family's ability to provide for the child's physical well-being. A colleague once asked me: "Taken the randomly selected infant or child from the entire world's population, what would be the most important question to ask?" That question is "Are you malnourished?" and in the great majority of cases, the tragic answer would be yes. To pursue the nuances of psychosexual development in these cases would be to suggest eating cake in the absence of bread. I will only say here that the evaluation must proceed in a hierarchical fashion and that the clinician must establish the hierarchy in each case.

The discussion of the four parameters of family function merits special notice. This is a new and relatively untested clinical tool. So far, systematic efforts to test the reliability of the four-dimensional model across clinicians have been unsuccessful. However, the results of using the model as a tool to teach something about the structure and function of families (and other groups) have been wonderful. In brief, one need only look for the crossover between anxiety and power. If one member of a dyad wields the power, the other member is anxious about it and the person in power is not, then the person in power is in control. In other words, a crossover of anxiety and power is a control point, and finding and exploring these control points can be the entirety of family therapy in some cases.

I suspect that the four-dimensional model of the family will be largely ignored. This is unfortunate. Learning to use it well requires systematic thinking through, in four-dimensional terms, of a number of cases. Students may be willing to do this, but the clinician who is already facile with one language will rarely bother to learn another.

One of my greatest interests is the usefulness of this four-dimensional analysis in larger social systems. My own bias is that there is no upper limit to the size of the group to which this tool can be applied. For example, does the evolution of the Warfare configuration apply at the international level? Analyzing the nature of conflict has made me recognize that conflict must be understood in terms of the configuration of the relationship between contesting parties rather than in terms of the intensity of the relationship. In other words, a devoutly religious, gentle, soft-spoken pair of Quakers may express a vigorous conflict through intraverbal nuance; but conflict is conflict just the same. If both parties are anxious and are engaged in a power struggle, if each believes that "I'm OK but you're a turkey [symptom carrier]," and if neither will make an accommodation, how does this dyad's basic configuration differ from the one between Israel and Syria? I invite discussion of this point.

In writing this book and in seeking to implement some of its tools in a clinical setting, I have learned much about the limitations of the teachings of the ivory tower. The specific deficit in my training was in the area of the cost-benefit ratio. Even worse, this deficit was never acknowledged. We were taught that the university hospital was the place where things were "done right," and we snickered at the LMD (local medical doctor) who botched things up. But we did not have the faintest notion about what the practice of medicine was like. Consider, for example, testing of hearing. If we wanted to set up a clinic to test the hearing of school children and if our budget was severely limited, we would want to know the error rate of the different testing devices in comparison to the cost. By gently rubbing one's fingers together behind a child's head and asking him to tell you when he hears the sound, obtains some idea about his hearing at zero cost in equipment. But what is the rate of error? Tuning forks increase the specificity of the stimulus. The cost goes up, but by how much does the error rate go down? A screening audiometer increases the cost by another order of magnitude, and full-scale audiometry in a sound-proof room by several more. How much is gained? We don't know. We know all about the structure and function of the hearing apparatus, but we don't know how to test its function most efficiently.

In medical school we "practiced medicine" outside a cost-analysis context. The expense that drove us was the expense to our self-esteem of endless one-upmanship. But this is not the practice of medicine; it is a sad variant called CYOA, or cover-your-own-ass medicine (the analogy to a personality disorder is obvious). When, on teaching rounds, does the attending physician ever considered the cost to the patient and his family of "another EEG", a major surgical procedure, or extensive psychotherapy? He does not consider it, and in not doing so raises a hothouse plant that will fare badly in the real world. Could it be that in many cases, the practice of medicine in a total sense requires decisions involving cost-benefit ratio at least as often as technical specifics?

What do I suggest? I hope that the construction of a multilevel problem-plan list will encourage others to consider available options in terms of cost-benefit ratio. I dare not hope that the staffs of university hospitals will refrain from snickering at clinicians who are faced with an entirely different set of problems.

Although one colleague's most vigorous criticism of this book is that it says too little about intervention, perhaps it actually says too much about intervention. In my opinion, we do not know much about intervention into complex systems. The different therapies tend to apply to special populations; we know little about the general case.

At last this project has reached a resting place. It can never be completed because development is a process. I welcome your comments, criticisms, and suggestions.

APPENDIX

The clinician needs a set of tools for day-to-day use. In some clinical settings, collection of a data base can be initiated by means of a questionnaire that is filled out before the first appointment, thus saving office time for the detailed pursuit of specific areas. In my own practice, I record standard data on forms such as those contained in this Appendix. Although this practice means that the first session is somewhat encumbered by the turning of pages and scribbling of notes, it has the distinct advantage of enabling me to obtain a fairly standard data base in written form by the end of the first hour. Businesslike note-taking does not necessarily impinge on the rapport that is so essential in an initial session; on the contrary, it can convey the message that because the child and family are important, we must carefully examine an adequate amount of data before making any recommendations.

Part A contains a questionnaire that is routinely given to parents before the initial interview. This questionnaire was written in collaboration with Andrea Lambert, R.N., M.S., who also assisted with the field trials.

Part B contains the intake evaluation form, which is filled out by the examiner during and after the initial interview with the identified patient and the parent or parents. This form undergoes constant modification and revision. A drawing of the family tree requires a separate sheet. The basic symbols will enable another clinician to read the drawing. The family tree should usually be accompanied by an explanatory paragraph. The level of differentiation, if necessary to understand the case, merits a separate heading and explanatory paragraph. Please do not use these forms as simple transplants. They are included here in the hope that they will facilitate the development of forms which are appropriate in other clinical settings.

A. Form Filled Out by Parent or Guardian

Your answers to the following questions will be of great value to the therapist who will be seeing you and your child. The information that you provide will be treated as *confidential information*. Please bring the completed form with you to your first interview. Thank you very much for your help.

Today's Date _____

GENERAL INFORMATION

Child's Name _____ Birthdate _____

Parents' (or guardians') names _____

Home Address _____ Home Telephone _____
               No.   Street

_____ Work Telephone _____
        City   State   Zip

Referring person or agency:

Address: _____ Telephone _____

Name of person completing this form and his relationship to child:

_____

Does mother and/or father live outside the home? If so, give address:

Is there or has there been any psychiatric/psychological counseling for anybody in the family? If so, who, when, and where?

Persons living in home where child lives:

Name	Relationship	Birth Date	Occupation or School and Grade	Employer
1.				
2.				
3.				
4.				
5.				
6.				
7.				
8.				

Is any other person important to the child or family (whether or not they are actual family members)?

II.   PRESENTING PROBLEM(S)

1. What is currently concerning you about your child or family?

2. When did the problem(s) start?

3. What happened that led you to come here?

4. What changes have you noticed in your family since this problem began?

5. Please list all professionals and agencies involved in the problem.

6. How has the child's problem been explained to you by other professionals?

7. What do parents see as needing change? (Please check.)
   _____ Child's behavior
   _____ Child's grades
   _____ Teacher's Attitude
   _____ School or school system

_____ Parent's expectations
_____ Child's personality
_____ Other (please describe)

8. Do both parents see the problem the same way?

9. What do you do about the problem at home?

10. Do both the school and parents see the problem the same way?

11. Does the child agree that there is a problem?

III. Have major changes of any kind occurred in your family in the last few years (for example: moves, changes in family composition, changes in income or situation, etc.)?

IV. SCHOOL

School Name_____ Phone_____

Address _____

Teacher _____

School Psychologist _____

School Counselor_____

Principal_____

1. Has the child had any difficulty going to school? (Describe.)

2. How important is it for the child to do well in school?

3. Did the child attend preschool?

4. Has the child been held back any grades? (Describe.)

5. Has the child been in special classes? (Describe.)

6. Has any psychological testing been done at school?

7. What does the child do well in at school?

8. What does the child do poorly in at school?

9. How does the child get along with other children in school?

10. How does the child get along with teachers, the principal, the counselor?

V. BROTHERS AND SISTERS, FRIENDS

1. How does child get along with brothers and sisters?

2. How does the child compare with brothers and sisters?

3. Friends
   a. Does child have friends in neighborhood?   yes___ no___
   b. Does child respond positively when approached?   yes___ no___
   c. Does child prefer adults to children?   yes___ no___
   d. One, two, or how many friends?
   e. Age of playmates preferred:

IV. RELATIONSHIPS WITH PARENTS

A. Child's relationship with father:
   1. Describe nature of contacts with father in home:

   2. Have there been separations?
      a. How old was child at time of separation?
      b. How often does father see child?
      c. Under what circumstances?

B. Child's relationship with mother:
   1. Describe nature of contacts with mother in home.

   2. Have there been separations?
      a. How old was child at time of separation?
      b. How often does mother see child?
      c. Under what circumstances?

C. Discipline:
   1. What kinds of things does child do that mother disciplines him for?

   2. What does she do about it?

   3. What kinds of things does child do that father disciplines him for?

   4. What does he do about it?

D. Feelings between parents and the child:
1. Do you like being with the child? (Elaborate.)

2. Do you find it difficult to be with the child? (Elaborate.)

3. What things do you most enjoy about the child?

4. What does the child do well?

VII.   MEDICAL

1. Child's doctor _____

   Address_____Telephone_____

2. List any serious accidents, including child's age and type of accident.

3. List all hospitalizations, operations and serious illnesses, including child's age and type of problem.

4. Is your child on any medications currently? If so, please list type and dosage, response, including side effects.

5. Has child received any medication in the past? What and when?

6. Is the child allergic to foods, medicines, house dust, animals, pollens? Anything else?

VIII.   LEGAL PROBLEMS

1. Has child ever been in trouble with the law?

2. If so, how many times?

3. Give approximate date(s):

4. What was the court's disposition?

5. Is the child currently on probation?

6. If yes, who is the probation officer?   Telephone _____

7. Is there any legal action currently pending?

IX.   MOOD AND TEMPERAMENT

a. Please check the answer that applies to the following questions about the child's *infancy:*

Behavior	Almost Never Applies	Does Not Usually Apply	Don't Know	Usually Applies	Almost Always Applies	Don't Understand the Question
1. Need a blanket-sleeper. Moved all around and kicked blankets off						
2. Ate, slept on an even schedule all by himself/herself						
3. Accepted new foods with no fuss						
4. Cheerful						
5. Handled a strange situation by moving toward it						
6. If he/she was going to cry, he/she would scream						
7. Would cry as soon as diaper was barely wet						
8. Repeatedly rejected water if he/she wanted milk						
9. Did not stop fussing even if comforted						
10. Overall, he/she was a difficult baby						
11. Overall, he/she was an easy baby						

b. Please check the answer that applies to the following questions about the *child's behavior now:*

Behavior	Almost Never Applies	Does Not Usually Apply	Don't Know	Usually Applies	Almost Always Applies	Don't Understand the Question
1. Always on the go						
2. Seems to run on an even schedule (waking, sleeping, eating)						
3. Adapts well to changes (new school, moving, etc.)						
4. Cheerful						
5. Handles a new situation by charging forward (new school, camp, etc.)						
6. He/she has no "middle range"; it's all or nothing.						
7. He/she is "hair trigger": little things are enough to set him/her off						
8. Has a long attention span						
9. Is easily distracted by any interference, however small						
10. Overall, he/she is a difficult child						
11. Overall, he/she is an easy child						
12. Overall, he/she is shy, but OK once he/she warms up						

X. DEVELOPMENTAL HiSTORY

    A. Pregnancy and delivery:

        1. Was the baby wanted?
           a. by mother?
           b. by father?

        2. Were there any marital or family problems at time of conception, pregnancy, and delivery?

    B. Mother's health during pregnancy:

        1. Health OK or not? Any problems?

        2. Did mother have prenatal care during this pregnancy?

        3. Diet OK?

        4. Was there any use of drugs, medications, alcohol?

        5. Was there any bleeding during the first three months of pregnancy?

    C. Delivery:

        1. Were there any difficulties with delivery?

        2. Was the baby OK at birth?
           Was the doctor concerned about the baby's health?
           Explain.

        3. Was an incubator or other special care given?
           How long?
           Describe:

        4. How much did the baby weigh at birth?

    D. Please give us your opinion of your child's development in the following areas. Was it slow, fast, or normal?

1. Physical development:

2. Development of language:

3. Development of intelligence:

4. Ability to relate to others:

5. Ability to appropriately experience and express feelings:

E. At what age did he/she

1. Walk alone?

2. Use single words?

3. Become toilet trained? Any difficulties? Explain.

B. Form Filled Out by Examiner

I. IDENTIFYING DATA

Names of

    Identified patient
    Mother
    Father
    Others in living unit

Address

Phone: home
      work
National Origin
Socioeconomic Level (of five)
    Identified patient:
    Age   years and   months
    Date of Birth
    Ordinal Position   of

School:
>
>   Name
>   Phone
>   Teacher
>   Grade
>   (Special placement?)

Referral Source:
>
>   Name
>   Phone

Previous therapists:
>
>   Name
>   Phone
>   Seen from   to

II. CLINICAL PROBLEM

A. Chief complaints:

Identified patient

Parents

School

Other

B. Duration and progression of the problem:

C. Major Life Changes:

D. Special Problems, (legal, medical, etc.):

III. TEMPERAMENTAL TYPE

| | *Describe by Parents* | | |
| *Trait* | *Infancy* | *Childhood* | *Currently Observed* |

Activity level

Adaptability

Rhythmicity

Mood

Approach/withdrawal

Intensity of reaction

Threshold

Persistence/attention
span

Distractibility

IV. CHILD'S DEVELOPMENTAL HISTORY

		Level		
Stage	*Biological*	*Psychological*	*Family*	*Social*
Prenatal (parental expectations)				
Pregnancy and delivery				
I. Infancy (basic trust vs. mistrust)				
II. Toddlerhood (autonomy vs. shame and doubt)				
III. Preschool (initiative vs. guilt)				
IV. Grade school (industry vs. inferiority)				

VI. FAMILY TREE

VII. FAMILY'S LEVEL OF DIFFERENTIATION (1–5)

VIII. PARAMETERS OF FAMILY FUNCTION

	Low	*High*
Anxiety		
Capacity to change		
Symptom-carrier role		
Power		

Summary of family dynamics:

IX. FORMULATION AND DIFFERENTIAL DIAGNOSIS:

Biological factors:

Developmental factors:

Diagnosis   Supporting data

Current situational factors:

Current coping maneuvers:

Differential diagnosis (GAP Report No. 62):

X. PROBLEM-PLAN LIST

Level	*Problem*	*Plan*
Biological		
Psychological		
Family		
Social		

REFERENCES

Ackerman, N. W. The emergence of family diagnosis and treatment: A personal view. *Psychotherapy*, 1967, **4**, 125–129.

Ackerman, N. W., & Behrens, M. L. Family diagnosis and clinical process. In S. Arieti (Ed.), *Handbook of American Psychiatry*. Vol. 2. New York: Basic Books, 1974.

Ackerman, N. W., & Sobel, R. Family diagnosis: An approach to the pre-school child. *American Journal of Orthopsychiatry*, 1950, **20**, 744–753.

Anastasi, A. *Psychological testing*. New York: Macmillan, 1968.

Anthony, E. J., & Koupernik, C. (Eds.). The impact of disease and death. Vol. 2. Anthony and Koupernik, *The child in his family*. New York: John Wiley & Sons, 1973.

Arieti, S. An overview of schizophrenia from a predominantly psychological approach. *American Journal of Psychiatry*, 1974, **131**, 241–249.

Barcai, A., & Rosenthal, M. K. Fears and tyranny: Observations on the tyrannical child. *Archives of General Psychiatry*, 1974, **30**, 392–395.

Beckett, J. A. General systems theory, psychiatry and psychotherapy. *International Journal of Group Psychotherapy*, 1973, **23**, 292–305.

Berne, E. *Games people play*. New York: Grove Press, 1964.

Boszormenyi-Nagy, I., & Spark, G. M. *Invisible loyalties*. New York: Harper & Row, 1973.

Bowen, M. The use of family theory in clinical practice. *Comprehensive Psychiatry*, 1966, **7**, 345–374.

Broman, S. H., Nichols, P. L., & Kennedy, W. A. *Preschool IQ: Prenatal and early developmental correlates.* New York: John Wiley & Sons, 1975.

Buckley, W. *Modern systems research for the behavioral scientist.* Chicago: Aldine, 1968.

Burns, R. C., & Kaufman, S. H. *Kinetic family drawings (K-F-D): Understanding children through kinetic drawings.* New York: Brunner/Mazel, 1970.

Buros, O. K. (Ed.). *Personality tests and reviews.* Highland Park, N.J.: Gryphon Press, 1970.

Campbell, D. T., & Stanley, J. *Experimental and quasi-experimental designs for research.* Chicago: Rand McNally, 1963.

Capek, M. *The philosophical impact of contemporary physics.* New York: Van Nostrand, 1961.

Cartwright, D. (Ed.). *Studies in social power.* Ann Arbor, Mich.: Institute for Social Research, 1959.

Chess, S. *An introduction to child psychiatry.* New York: Grune & Stratton, 1969.

Coddington, R. D. The significance of life events as etiologic factors in the diseases of children. I. A survey of professional workers. *Journal of Psychosomatic Research*, 1972, **16**, 7–18. (a)

Coddington, R. D. The significance of life events as etiologic factors in the diseases of children. II. A study of a normal population. *Journal of Psychosomatic Research*, 1972, **16**, 205–213. (b).

Committee on Nomenclature and Statistics, American Psychiatric Association. *DSM-II: Diagnostic and statistical manual of mental disorders.* (2nd ed.) Washington, D.C.: American Psychiatric Association, 1968.

Commoner, B. *The closing circle.* New York: Alfred A. Knopf, 1971.

Cytryn, L., & McKnew, D. H. Proposed classification of childhood depression. *American Journal of Psychiatry*, 1972, **129**, 149–155.

Ellis, A., & Harper, R. A. *A guide to rational living.* North Hollywood, Calif.: Hal Leighton, 1961.

Engel, G. L. A life setting conducive to illness: The giving-up-given-up complex. *Annals of Internal Medicine*, 1968, **69**, 293–300.

Erikson, E. *Childhood and society.* New York: W. W. Norton, 1950.

Ferreira, A. J. Family myth and homeostasis. *Archives of General Psychiatry*, 1963, **9**, 457–463.

Fish, B. Contributions of developmental research to a theory of schizophrenia. In J. Hellmuth (Ed.), *Exceptional infant.* Vol. 2 *Studies in Abnormalities.* New York: Brunner/ Mazel, 1971.

Flavell, J. H. *The developmental psychology of Jean Piaget.* New York: Van Nostrand Reinhold, 1963.

Forrester, J. W. *Principles of systems.* Cambridge, Mass.: Wright-Allen Press, 1968.

Framo, J. L. Symptoms from a family transactional viewpoint. *International Psychiatry Clinics,* 1970, **7,** 125–171.

Frankenburg, W. K., & Dodds, J. B. The Denver developmental screening test. *Journal of Pediatrics,* 1967, **2,** 181–191.

French, A. P., & Steward, M. S. Adaptation and affect: Toward a synthesis of Piagetian and psychoanalytic psychologies. *Perspectives in Biology and Medicine,* 1975, **18,** 464–474.

French, A. P., & Steward, M. S. Family dynamics, childhood depression, and attempted suicide in a 7-year-old boy: A case study. *Suicide,* 1975, **5,** 29–37.

Gardner, R. A. *Therapeutic communication with children: The mutual storytelling technique.* New York: Science House, 1971.

Gardner, R. A. *Techniques of child psychotherapy.* Fort Lee, N.J.: Behavioral Sciences Tape Library, 1972.

Geselle, A., & Amatruda, C. S. *Developmental diagnosis.* New York: Hoeber Medical Division, Harper & Row, 1947.

Glaser, K. Masked depression in children and adolescents. *American Journal of Psychotherapy,* 1967, **21,** 565–574.

Goodman, J., & Sours, J. *The child mental status examination.* New York: Basic Books, 1967.

Gray, W., & Rizzo, N. D. History and development of general system theory. In W. Gray, F. J. Duhl, & Rizzo (Eds.), *General system theory and psychiatry.* Boston: Little, Brown, 1969.

Grinker, R. R., Sr. *Psychiatry in broad perspective.* New York: Behavioral Publications, 1975.

Group for the Advancement of Psychiatry. *Psychopathological disorders in childhood: Theoretical considerations and a proposed classification.* Report No. 62. New York: Author, 1966. (This report can be obtained from the Group for the Advancement of Psychiatry, 419 Park Avenue South, New York, N.Y. 10016.)

Haley, J. Research on family patterns: An instrument measure. *Family Process,* 1964, **3,** 41–65.

Haley, J. Speech sequence of normal and abnormal families with two children present. *Family Process,* 1967, **6,** 81–97.

Hall, A. D., & Fagen, R. G. Definition of system. In W. Buckley (Ed.), *Modern systems research for the behavioral scientist.* Chicago: Aldine, 1968.

Hall, C. S., & Lindzey, G. *Theories of personality.* New York: John Wiley & Sons, 1970.

Harris, D. B. *Childrens' drawings as measures of intellectual maturity: A revision and extension of the Goodenough Draw-A-Man test.* New York: Harcourt, Brace & World, 1964.

Hoffman, P. J., Slovic, P., & Rorer, L. G. An analysis-of-variance model for the assessment of configural cue utilization in clinical judgment. *Psychological Bulletin,* 1968, **69,** 338–349.

Hollingshead, A. B., & Redlich, F. C. *Social classes and mental illness.* New York: John Wiley & Sons, 1958.

Hoover, C. F., & Franz, J. D. Siblings in the families of schizophrenics. *Archives of General Psychiatry,* 1972, **26,** 334–342.

Hurst, J. W., & Walker, H. K. (Eds.) *The problem-oriented system.* New York: Medcom Press, 1972.

Ilg, F. L., & Ames, L. B. *School readiness.* Cleveland: Harper & Row, 1964.

Inglis, B. J. *A history of medicine.* New York: World Publishing, 1965.

Johnson, A. Sanctions for superego lacunae of adolescents. In K. R. Eissler (Ed.), *Searchlights on delinquency.* New York: International Universities Press, 1949.

Johnson, D. M. *Systematic introduction to the psychology of thinking.* New York: Harper & Row, 1972.

Kahneman, D., & Tversky, A. On the psychology of prediction. *Psychological Review,* 1973, **80,** 237–251.

Kohlberg, L. Early education: A cognitive developmental view. *Child Development,* 1968, **39,** 1013–1062.

Laughlin, C. D., & D'Aquili, C. G. *Biogenetic structuralism.* New York: Columbia University Press, 1974.

Lidz, T., Cornelison, A., Fleck, S., & Terry, D. Intrafamilial environment of schizophrenic patients. II. Marital schism and marital stew. *American Journal of Psychiatry,* 1957, **114** 241–248.

Lenneberg, G. H. On explaining language: The development of language may best be understood in the context of developmental biology. *Science,* 1969, **164,** 635–643.

Long, N. J., & Morse, W. C. *Conflict in the classroom.* Belmont, Calif.: Wadsworth, 1965.

Mahler, M. *On human symbiosis and the vicissitudes of individuation.* New York: International Universities Press, 1968.

Malmquist, C. P. Depressions in childhood and adolescence. *New England Journal of Medicine,* 1971, **281,** 887–893 and 955–961.

Mazur, W. P. (Ed.). *The problem-oriented system in the psychiatric hospital: A manual for mental health professionals.* Garden Grove, Calif.: Trainex Press, 1974.

McDermott, J. F., & Char, W. F. The undeclared war between child and family therapy. *Journal of the American Academy of Child Psychiatry,* 1974, **13,** 422–436.

Meehl, P. *Clinical versus statistical prediction: A theoretical analysis and a review of the evidence.* Minneapolis, Minn.: University of Minnesota Press, 1954.

Meehl, P. Why I do not attend case conferences. In Meehl, *Psycho diagnosis: Selected papers.* Minneapolis: University of Minnesota Press, 1973.

Mendell, D., & Fisher, S. An approach to neurotic behavior in terms of a three generation family model. *Journal of Nervous and Mental Disease,* 1956, **123,** 171–180.

Menninger, K. A. *A manual for psychiatric case study.* New York: Grune & Stratton, 1962.

Menninger, K. A., Mayman, M., & Pruyser, P. *The vital balance.* New York: Viking Press, 1963.

Minuchin, S. *Families and family therapy.* Cambridge, Mass.: Harvard University Press, 1974.

Mishler, E., & Wexler, N. Family interaction process and schizophrenia. *International Journal of Psychiatry,* 1966, **2,** 375–430.

Mussen, P. H. (Ed.). *Carmichael's manual of child psychology.* New York: John Wiley & Sons, 1970.

Mutti, M., Sterling, H. M., Spalding, N. V., & Crawford, C. S. *QNST: Quick neurological screening test.* San Rafael, Calif.: Academic Therapy Publications, 1974.

Nagera, H. *Monograph series of the psycho analytic study of the child.* Vol. 2. New York: International Universities Press, 1966.

Niswander, K. R., & Gordon, M. *The Collaborative Study: The women and their pregnancies.* Philadelphia: W. B. Saunders, 1972.

Niswander, K. R., Gordon, M., & Drage, J. S. The effect of intrauterine hypoxia on the child surviving to 4 years. *American Journal of Obstetrics and Gynecology,* 1975, **121,** 892.

Panzetta, A. F. Toward a scientific psychiatric nosology: Conceptual and pragmatic issues. *Archives of General Psychiatry,* 1974, **30,** 154–161.

Piaget, J. *The origins of intelligence in children.* New York: W. W. Norton, 1963.

Piaget, J. Piaget's theory. In P. H. Mussen (Ed.), *Carmichael's handbook of child psychology.* New York: John Wiley & Sons, 1970.

Piaget, J. Some aspects of operations. In M. W. Piers (Ed.), *Play and development.* New York: Van Nostrand, 1972.

Piaget, J. *Structuralism.* New York: Harper & Row, 1971.

Piaget, J., & Inhelder, B. *The psychology of the child.* New York: Basic Books, 1969.

Piers, M. W. (Ed.). *Play and development.* New York: W. W. Norton, 1975.

Reusch, J. Synopsis of the theory of human communication. *Psychiatry: Journal for the Study of Interpersonal Processes,* 1953, **16,** 215–243.

Satir, V. M. *Conjoint family therapy.* Palo Alto, Calif.: Science & Behavior Books, 1967.

Satir, V. M. Symptomatology: A family production. In J. G. Howells (Ed.), *Theory and practice of family psychiatry.* New York: Brunner/Mazel, 1971.

Santostefano, S. Cognitive controls vs. cognitive styles: An approach to diagnosing and treating cognitive disabilities in children. *Seminars in Psychiatry,* 1969, **1,** 291–317.

Scagliotta, G. G. *Initial learning assessment.* San Rafael, Calif.: Academic Therapy Publications, 1970.

Schopler, E., & Luftin, J. Thought disorders in parents of psychotic children: A function of test anxiety. *Archives of General Psychiatry,* 1969, **20,** 174–181.

Silver, L. *Social and emotional difficulties of children with learning disabilities.* New York: John Wiley & Sons, in press.

Silver, L. B. The playroom diagnostic evaluation of children with neurologically based learning disabilities. *Journal of the American Academy of Child Psychiatry,* 1976, **15,** 240.

Simmons, J. E. *Psychiatric evaluation of children.* Philadelphia: Lea & Febiger, 1969.

Stallknecht, N. P., & Brumbaugh, R. S. *The spirit of western philosophy.* New York: Longmans, Green, 1950.

Szurek, S. Genesis of psychopathic personality traits. *Psychiatry,* 1942, **5,** 1–6.

Thomas, A., Chess, S., & Birch, H. G. The origin of personality. *Scientific American,* 1970, **223,** 102–109.

Thorndike, R. L., & Hagen, E. Measurement and evaluation in psychology and education. New York: John Wiley & Sons, 1955.

Toman, W. *Family constellation: Its effects on personality and social behavior.* New York: Springer Publishing, 1969.

Tseng, W.-S., Arensdorf, A. M., McDermott, J. F., Hansen, M. J., & Fukunaga, C. S. Family diagnosis and classification. *Journal of the American Academy of Child Psychiatry,* 1976, **15,** 15–35.

Von Bertalanffy, L. *General system theory.* New York: George Braziller, 1968.

Waddington, C. H. New patterns in genetics and development. New York: Columbia University Press, 1962.

Watzlawick, P., Bleavin, J., & Jackson, D. *Pragmatics of human communication.* New York: W. W. Norton, 1967.

Weed, L. L. Quality control. In H. K. Walker, J. W. Hurst & M. F. Woody (Eds.), *Applying the problem-oriented system.* New York: Medcom Press, 1973.

Weed, L. L. The problem-oriented record. In J. W. Hurst & H. K. Walker (Eds.), *The problem-oriented system.* New York: Medcom Press, 1975.

Wender, P. H. *Minimal brain dysfunction in children.* New York: Wiley-Interscience, 1971.

Werner, E. F. *Keiki A Opio: Kauai's children come of age.* Honolulu: University of Hawaii Press, 1976.

Werner, E. F., Bierman, J. M., & French, F. E. *The children of Kauai: A longitudinal study from the prenatal period to age ten.* Honolulu: University of Hawaii Press, 1971.

Wolff, S. The contribution of obstetric complications to the etiology of behavior disorders in childhood. *Journal of Child Psychology and Psychiatry,* 1967, **8,** 57–66.

Woody, M. F. *Applying the problem-oriented system.* In Hurst, J. W., & Walker, H. K. *The problem-oriented system.* New York: Medcom Press, 1973.

BIBLIOGRAPHY

The following sources provide a good beginning for any search of the literature in child psychiatry.

Berlin, I. N. (Eds.) *Bibliography of child psychiatry.* Official publication of the American Academy of Child Psychiatry. New York: Human Sciences Press, 1976.

Chess, S., & Thomas, A. (Eds.). *Annual progress in child psychiatry and child development* Vols. 1–8. New York: Brunner/Mazel, 1968–1975.

Howells, J. G. (Ed.). *Modern perspectives in psychiatry.* New York: Brunner/Mazel, 1971. (This series contains three volumes of special interest: Vol. 1, *Modern perspectives in child psychiatry;* Vol. 3, *Modern perspectives in international child psychiatry;* and Vol. 4, *Modern perspectives in adolescent psychiatry.*)

Olson, D. H., & Dahl, N. S. *Inventory of marriage and family literature. Minneapolis: University of Minnesota Press, 1975.*

INDEX